Zoltan Rona MD

Osteoarthritis

Treat and reverse joint pain naturally

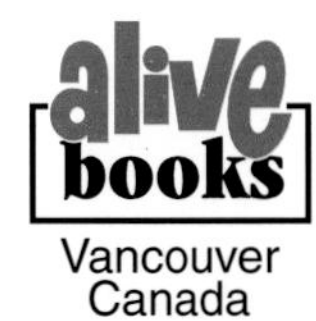

Vancouver
Canada

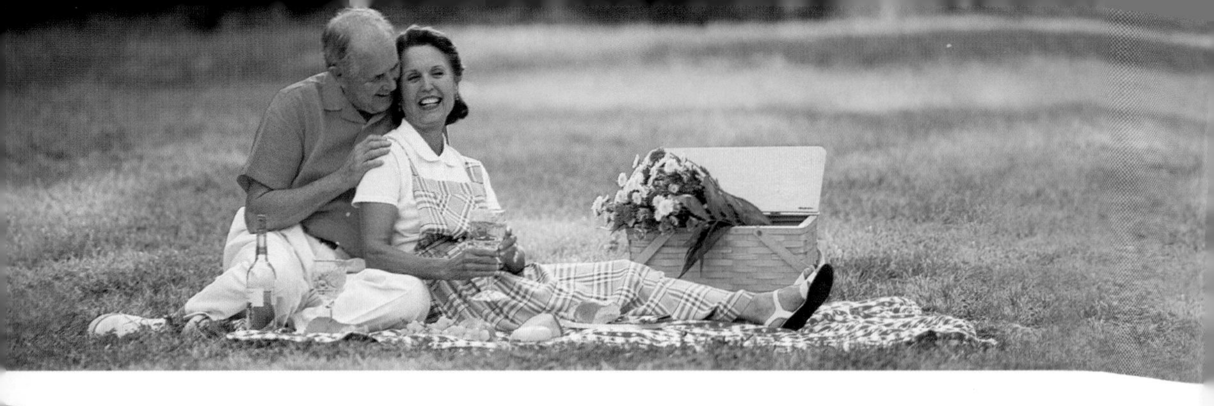

Contents

All About Osteoarthritis

Introduction 6
Understanding Arthritis 8
Osteoarthritis 10
The Importance of Cartilage 12
What Causes Osteoarthritis? 13
Hydrochloric Acid Deficiency 14
Vitamin D Deficiency 14
Fluoride 14
Mineral Deficiencies 15
Food Allergies 15
Conventional Treatments 16
Treating and Reversing Osteoarthritis 17
Exercise and Physical Therapy 17
Weight Loss 17
Diet 17
Food Allergy and Lab Tests 19
Supplements 22

Note: Conversions in this book (from imperial to metric) are not exact. They have been rounded to the nearest measurement for convenience. Exact measurements are given in imperial. The recipes in this book are by no means to be taken as therapeutic. They simply promote the philosophy of both the author and *alive* books in relation to whole foods, health, and nutrition, while incorporating the practical advice given by the author in the first section of the book.

Healthy Recipes

Healthy Start Breakfast 38
Pink Grapefruit and Avocado Salad 40
Baby Romaine with Tropical Fruit 42
Watercress Salad with Lentils 44
Corn and Avocado Soup 46
Green Pea Soup with Polenta Dumplings 48
Ruben Sandwich with Roasted Yam 50
Currant Rice with Curried Vegetables 52
Vegetarian Paella 54
Panfried Polenta with Vegetable Ragout 56
Apricot-Rice Patty with Fresh Fruit 58
Cream of Wheat with Fresh Fruit 60

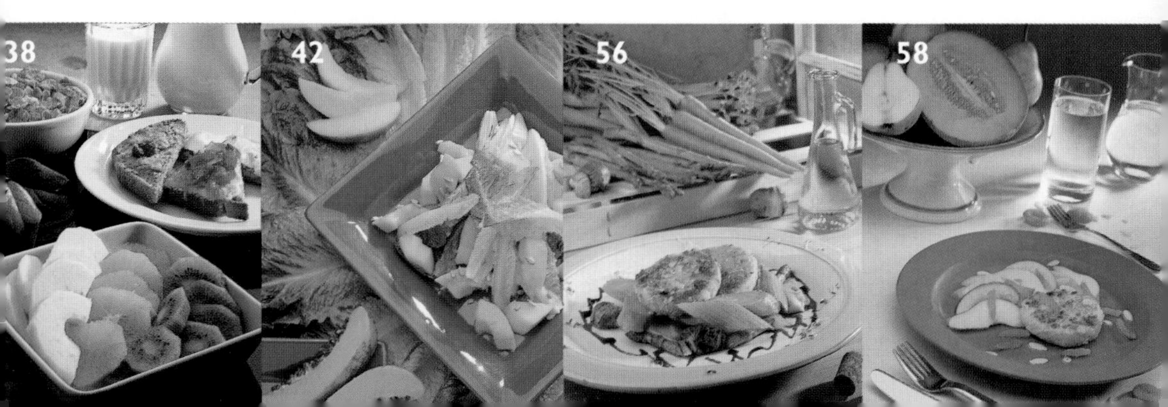

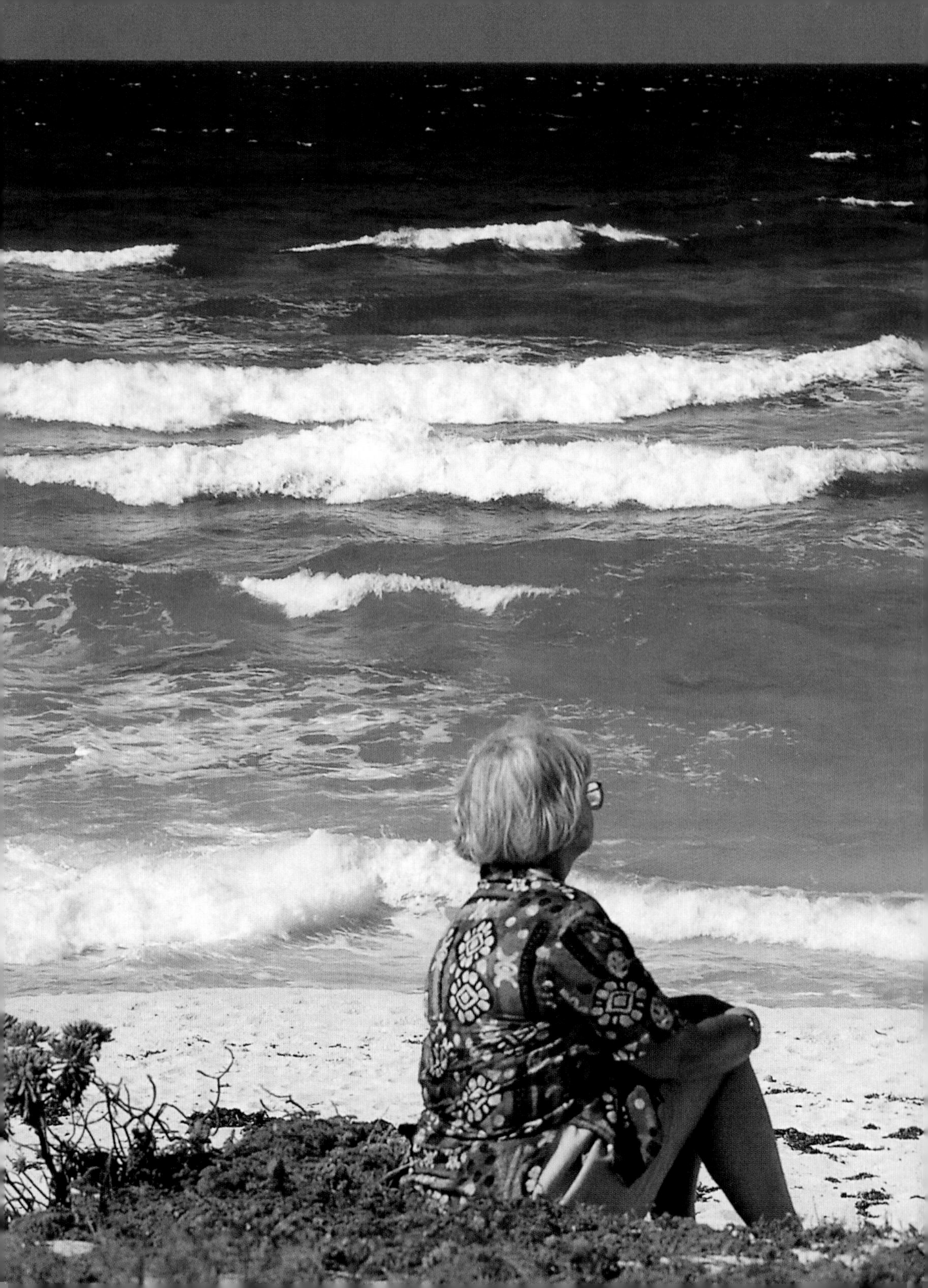

All About Osteoarthritis

I have had the opportunity to witness hundreds of people reverse or improve osteoarthritis naturally. – Zoltan Rona, MD

Most people, including doctors, are of the belief that arthritis is incurable, and that its symptoms can only be suppressed with drugs. Nothing could be further from the truth.

Introduction

Modern medicine has a great deal to offer when addressing acute illnesses or accidents. I know that if I were ever in a motor vehicle accident, resulting in the steering wheel of my dashboard stuck into my chest cavity, that I would want the best of what conventional medicine and surgery has to offer to save my life. Unfortunately, I cannot say the same about the value and effectiveness of modern medicine in its approach to dealing with chronic degenerative diseases such as osteoarthritis.

NSAIDS

Nonsteroidal anti-inflammatory drugs, or NSAIDS, are the most common of the conventional treatment approaches for osteoarthritis. They are also the most damaging, causing gastrointestinal bleeding and ulcers, and in some cases, potentially serious liver problems. These drugs do offer short-term pain relief but they inhibit cartilage repair. Given that healthy cartilage is an important factor in preventing osteoarthritis, NSAIDS, in the long run, will prove to worsen, not help, arthritis.

You are, no doubt, reading this book because medical treatments have failed to relieve the signs and symptoms of osteoarthritis. Perhaps you are taking prescription drugs with too many side effects and not enough pain relief; and you are taking these drugs with no end in sight. Or perhaps you have a friend or loved one crippled with the problem, awaiting knee or hip replacement surgery, barely getting through the day with worsening pain and stomach ulcers from the drug prescriptions.

Whatever your situation, I can just about guarantee you that medical or surgical approaches to the problem will never address the cause or source of the damage, just the pain. And that's if you're one of the lucky ones. In fact, most medical treatments, in particular the hugely popular prescription and over-the-counter NSAIDS (non-steroidal anti-inflammatory drugs) make the disease worse by interfering with cartilage repair. Aside from that, long-term use of NSAIDS has been linked to ulcer development, blood loss from hemorrhage and death.

A few years ago, Evelyn (not her real name), a woman in her late fifties, came to see me because years of prescription painkillers and NSAIDS had failed to relieve jaw, neck and back pain diagnosed by her family doctor and specialists as osteoarthritis. She told me that she didn't believe in vitamins or alternative medicine and only consulted me at the urgings of several of her friends who had been able to get rid of their arthritis using some of my suggestions. "If you can help me get rid of this pain, it will be a miracle," were her desperate words on her first office visit.

Three months later, with the diet changes and some of the natural supplements you are about to read about in this book, Evelyn was not only pain-free but free of medications and playing golf again with her friends. Her family doctor and arthritis specialist, unfortunately, believe that Evelyn's recovery was in her head ("the placebo effect"). As you are about to read, however, scientific studies prove otherwise.

Osteoarthritis is reversible. At the very least, the signs and symptoms can be arrested and the discomforts improved.

The good news you are about to read about in this book, is that osteoarthritis is reversible. At the very least, the signs and symptoms can be arrested and the discomforts improved enough to allow better joint function. While you will read about the newly popular natural remedies like glucosamine sulfate, chondroitin sulfate, essential fatty acids, niacinamide and others, you will also learn about the kind of diet to follow to both prevent and reverse osteoarthritis.

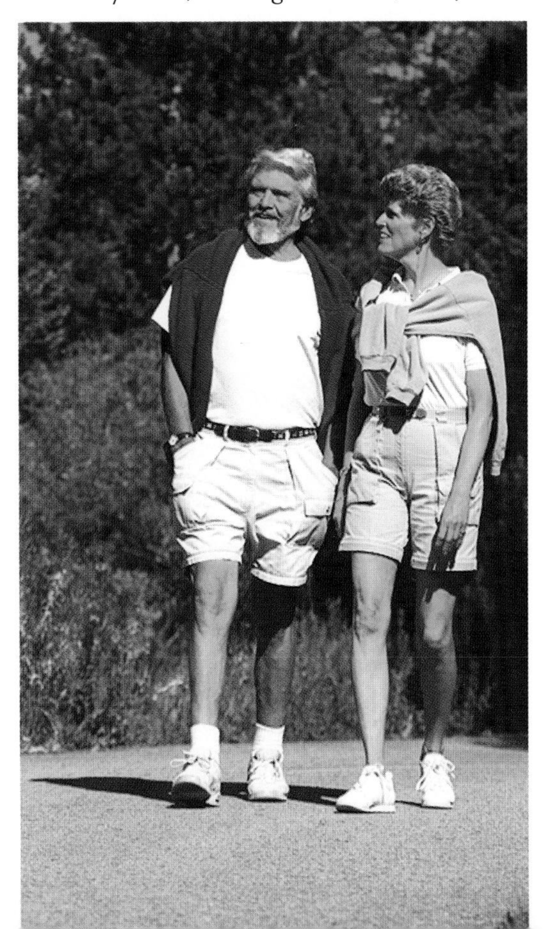

In nearly 23 years of medical practice, I have had the opportunity to witness hundreds of people reverse or improve osteoarthritis naturally. The following pages will help you take advantage of the latest scientific knowledge about natural remedies and my clinical experience helping people overcome a truly annoying, painful and distressing, yet reversible, condition.

Common Types of Arthritis and Arthritic Conditions	
Ankylosing spondylitis	Osteoporosis
Back pain	Polyarteritis
Carpal tunnel syndrome	Polymyalgia rheumatica
Degenerative joint disease	Psoriatic arthritis
Fibromyalgia	Reiter's syndrome
Gout	Rheumatoid arthritis
Juvenile rheumatoid arthritis	Scleroderma
Lyme disease	Sjogren's syndrome
Systemic Lupus erythematosus	

About 50 million North Americans (approximately one out of seven people) have arthritis. Of this number, at least 30 million are women, and nearly 300,000 are children under age eighteen. According to various arthritis foundations and other experts, in another 20 years, as baby boomers grow older and people live longer in general, close to 70 million people in Canada and the United States will have arthritis.

Rheumatoid Arthritis

Rheumatoid arthritis is a more destructive form of arthritis than osteoarthritis, as it can cause crippling and deformation at an early age. The true cause of this disease is unknown. However, it is known that it belongs to a family of autoimmune diseases in which the body attacks its own tissues as a result of an immune system reaction. Some other facts about rheumatoid arthritis are as follows:

- It is common in people under 40 and children.
- Juvenile rheumatoid arthritis is six times more common in girls as boys.
- This disease affects about three million people in Noth America.
- Common symptoms are stiffness, anemia, fatigue, weight loss, fever and severe pain.
- It is often associated with physical or emotional stress, poor nutrition and bacterial infections.

To understand how to reverse rheumatoid arthritis naturally, one must understand how to properly treat autoimmune diseases in general. For more information read the *alive* Natural Health Guide dedicated to this topic.

Arthritis is a general term applied to any inflammation of a joint. There are more than one hundred conditions that are currently identified by this term. Some of them–osteoarthritis,

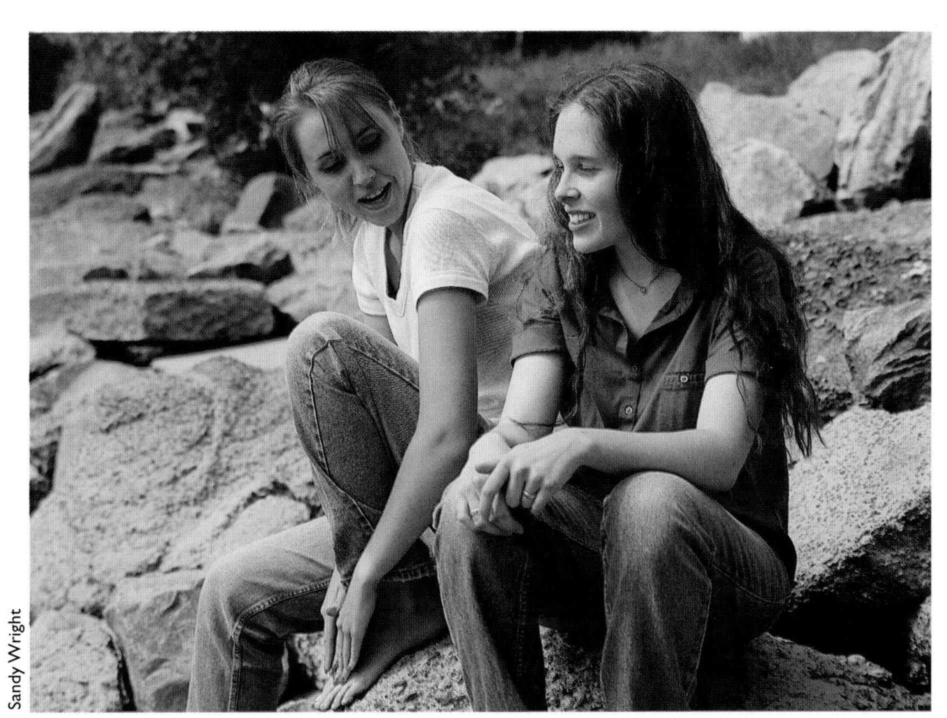

Sandy Wright

There are more than one hundred conditions that are currently identified as arthritis, affecting people of all ages.

for example–can be relatively mild; other forms like rheumatoid arthritis and ankylosing spondylitis can become crippling. Arthritis may even be a feature of life-threatening systemic illnesses such as lupus.

Arthritis is not necessarily a modern disease; there is considerable archeological evidence for its existence in prehistoric man, Egyptian mummies and virtually every human culture ever studied. What is most noticeable about the disease in North America in the year 2000 is the growing number of people of all ages suffering from one form or another.

Most people, including doctors, are of the belief that arthritis is incurable, and that its symptoms can only be suppressed with drugs. Nothing could be further from the truth. Arthritis of any kind can be arrested and, in most cases, reversed. If one provides the body with an optimal diet and supplemental nutrients, even the most crippling forms of arthritis can get better. Moreover, this is an increasingly common observation that has been the subject of many scientific and medical journal publications.

Osteoarthritis

The signs and symptoms of osteoarthritis are most often noticed gradually, over a period of several years.

Osteoarthritis is the most common form of joint disease, and is generally considered to be due to "wear and tear" of the joints, which leads to damage of the joint surfaces and pain on movement. Osteoarthritis tends to run in families, and three times as many women contract the disease as men. Although generally rare before age forty, nearly everyone has some degree of osteoarthritis by age sixty. Many people with osteoarthritis have mild or no symptoms, and are only made aware they have the condition in the course of x-rays done for other diagnostic reasons.

Osteoarthritis ...
• Is rare before age 40 and very common after age 60.
• Affects at least 16 million people in Canada and the US.
• Runs in families.
• Affects three times as many women as men.
• Is related to the wear and tear of joints through aging.
• May be mild, showing up only on x-rays.
• Is sometimes caused by an injury or defect in the protein part of cartilage.
• Involves deterioration of the cartilage that covers the ends of the bone.

Symptoms of Osteoarthritis

One might first notice a stiffness in the joints upon arising each day. This stiffness worsens over time, eventually causing pain that is relieved only by strong analgesic drugs. Sports and other strenuous physical activity must be curtailed, and long periods of time spent resting or relaxing are needed to fully alleviate the pain. Sound familiar? Such are the early signs and symptoms of osteoarthritis, common to even the fittest members of our population.

The different types of arthritis have their own set of characteristic signs, symptoms and course, and the way in which the disease progresses also varies from individual to individual. However, just about anyone suffering from arthritis will, at some point, experience pain and limited movement at certain sites along the body. While most types of arthritis are chronic, in many cases the symptoms come and go. There will be times when the disease is active (flares) and times when it is inactive (in remission). Depending on the severity of the specific type, arthritis can interfere with even the most ordinary activities of living, such as walking, dressing or bathing.

Osteoarthritis causes pain, swelling, stiffness and limited mobility of any given joint with activity. These signs and symptoms are most often noticed gradually, over a period of several years. They are also highly variable in the degree of intensity from person to person. For example, x-rays may show the presence of Heberden's nodes (a flaring of the ends of the bones resembling a bump on a log) but the person may not notice any pain or stiffness. In another individual with a smaller flaring of the bones, be it in the knees or the spinal vertebrae, the pain and stiffness may be so excruciating that mobility is completely suppressed.

In my practice I have noticed many people in their sixties and seventies with enlarged knuckles and finger joints caused by osteoarthritis who do not complain of pain or have any degree of discomfort or loss of joint ranges of motion. On the other hand, an equal number may be in such pain that handwriting or typing is not possible.

In most cases stiffness and limited range of motion are more severe in the morning or on certain days. In fact, some arthritis sufferers can predict, with great accuracy, changes in the weather: They feel it in their bones, so to speak, as their symptoms flare with changes in barometric pressure. Pain and the other symptoms of osteoarthritis tend to get worse with activity so

Arthritis is a disease that, without concerted effort and treatment, lasts a lifetime.

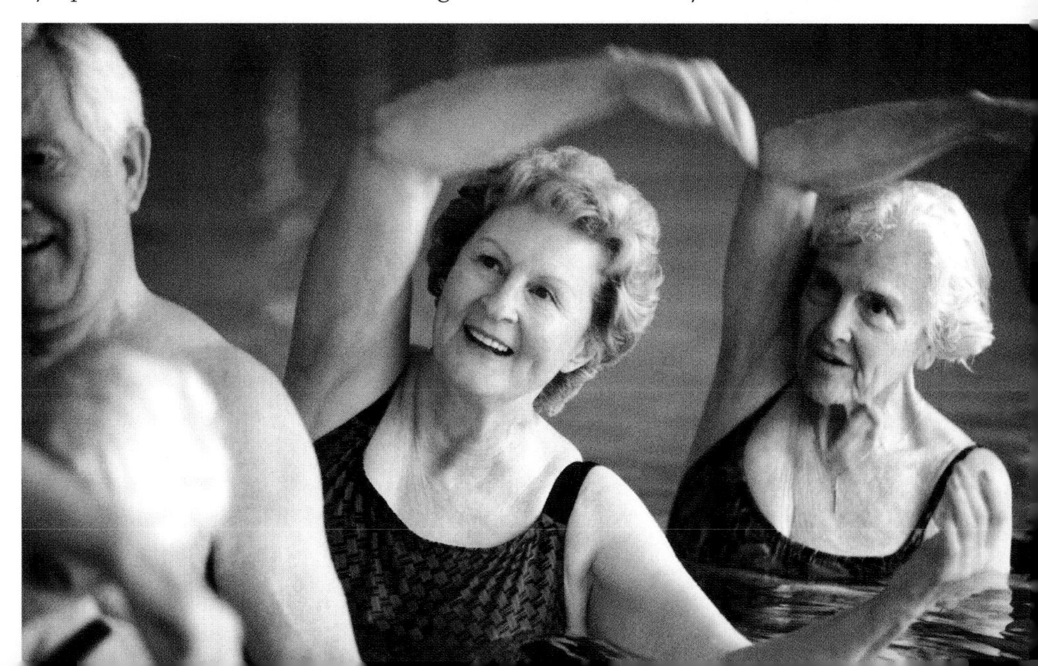

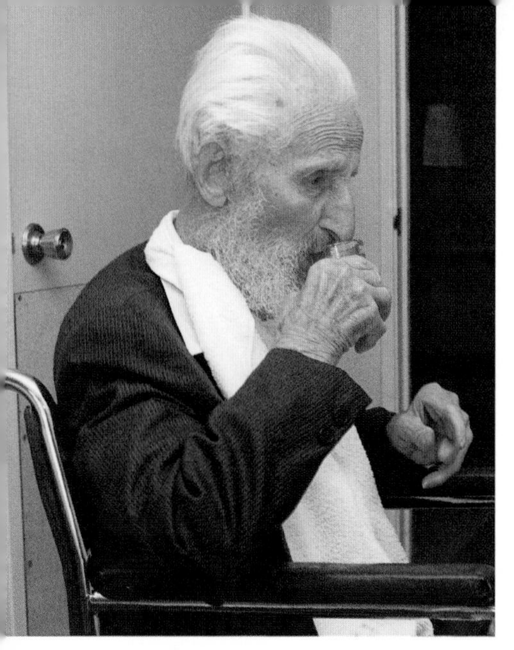

Osteoarthritis causes pain, swelling, stiffness and limited mobility.

that the end of the day is the worst time for most osteoarthritis sufferers.

In the later stages of osteoarthritis the victim eventually develops inflammation (redness, heat, swelling, pain) and enlargement of the joint. Muscle contractures (severe tightening) and spasms may occur, and joint mobility becomes progressively impaired. Commonly, there is a hard, bony swelling of the joints, and a gritty feeling (or even noise) when the joint is moved, a characteristic called *crepitus*. In the final stages of osteoarthritis, the joint becomes unrecognizable and is held in a virtually fused position.

Sometimes, for unknown reasons, symptoms disappear completely for considerable stretches of time, only to flare up again later. Arthritis is a disease that, without concerted effort and treatment, lasts a lifetime. What may be the best kept secret about the disease, however, is that the signs and symptoms can be reversed by using the natural methods discussed in this book.

The Importance of Cartilage

The major concern with osteoarthritis is degeneration of the articular cartilage that covers the ends of the bones. The integrity of cartilage appears to be the most important factor in the prevention of osteoarthritis. Cartilage deteriorates due to heredity, the wear and tear of daily living, injuries, excess weight, repetitive stress on a joint as well as various nutritional imbalances.

Joints like the knee, knuckle, wrist, elbow, shoulder, hip and ankle are cushioned by cartilage and a pad-like sac or cavity called the bursa, which is lined with the synovial membrane. This inner lining produces the synovial fluid that keeps the joints lubricated. Ligaments, a network of fibrous tissue, connect and support the components that comprise the joint.

Repetitive stress and strain on the joints (wear and tear) eventually exceeds their ability to recover, at which point an inflammatory process sets in. Inflammation–a natural part of the body's response to injury and infection–produces swelling, pain, warmth and redness. When inflammation is persistent, intense or recurrent, it leads to stiffness, rigidity and tissue damage.

Pain, the body's signal that something is wrong, occurs as the joint is moved to the brink of its limits. With arthritis, mobility decreases and the muscles surrounding the joint weaken, allowing further injury to the joint. With time, the cartilage breaks down, the bone erodes and the joints become deformed. The normally smooth sliding surfaces of the bones become jagged and irregular. With complete cartilage deterioration, bone rubs against bone. Bone spurs or osteophytes (flaring) may form around the joint in response to this loss of cartilage.

The integrity of cartilage appears to be the most important factor in the prevention of osteoarthritis.

Cartilage and Osteoarthritis

Cartilage is the fibrous connective tissue that supports the skeleton at specific sites throughout the body. It forms the temporary skeletal system of the fetus and infant but is gradually replaced by bones as the body matures. The cartilage that remains into adulthood is found mainly in the joints, where it reduces friction and gives flexibility. Cartilage is composed of collagen, a protein that is also found in skin, ligaments, tendons and bones. With osteoarthritis, the cartilage that covers the ends of the bones breaks down, and the normally smooth surfaces of the bones become jagged and irregular, with accompanying pain and discomfort. To prevent the development of arthritis it is essential that the integrity of the cartilage be maintained.

Once this has occurred, the later stages of osteoarthritis involve the tendons, ligaments and muscles that hold the joint together. These supporting structures get weakened, leading to joint deformity, pain and worsening stiffness. The bones become more brittle and there is an increased risk of fractures. Regardless of the cause, this is the process by which arthritis develops.

What Causes Osteoarthritis?

Many factors determine whether a joint develops osteoarthritis, including a family history of the condition and previous damage to the joint through injury or surgery. Although osteoarthritis is generally considered to be one of the consequences of aging, people who have suffered from various athletic injuries

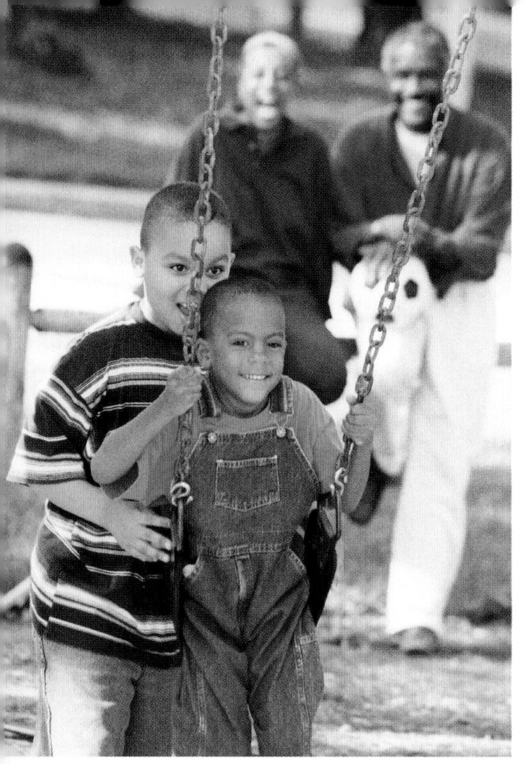

in their twenties or thirties (e.g., torn knee cartilage) frequently develop osteoarthritis in the injured joints well before their forties.

Hydrochloric acid deficiency is yet another potential cause of osteoarthritis; such a deficiency may be present in up to 40 percent of patients with arthritis. Low levels of stomach acidity prevent complete protein digestion. The undigested polypeptides are absorbed, eliciting allergic reactions that can lead to joint inflammation as well as inflammation in other tissues and organs.

Moreover, since a healthy level of stomach acidity is required for mineral absorption, low levels of hydrochloric acid may be responsible for malabsorption of minerals like copper, zinc, manganese, calcium and magnesium. These minerals are important for healthy bone metabolism; thus, a deficiency can make osteoarthritis worse.

Vitamin D deficiency can also lead to osteoarthritis. Vitamin D assists the body in the absorption of calcium, and has been used for the treatment and prevention of osteoporosis (bone thinning due to demineralization). Low vitamin D intake and blood levels are associated with an increased risk for the progression of osteoarthritis.

Low blood levels of vitamin D are also related to loss of cartilage and degenerative bony spur formation. Dr. Timothy E. McAlindon and associates studied 556 patients (with an average age of seventy years) and found that the risk of progression of osteoarthritis of the knee for participants that had low vitamin D intake and blood levels was three times that of those without these deficiencies. Patients with osteoarthritis who have modest vitamin D intake or low blood levels may benefit from increased vitamin D intake or sunlight exposure.

Fluoride may also cause osteoarthritis. At levels as low as one part-per-million (PPM) in drinking water, fluoride gives rise to an increase in the urine concentration of certain biological chemicals that signal the breakdown of collagen as well as the irregular formation of collagen in the body.

Collagen is important, making up more than 30 percent of the protein in the body. It serves as the major structural component of skin, ligaments, tendons, muscles, cartilage, bones and teeth. Fluoride disruption of the nature of collagen in the body results in premature wrinkling of the skin, weakening of ligaments, stiffness of the joints and arthritis.

Mineral deficiencies can either cause or worsen osteoarthritis. Calcium, magnesium, zinc, copper, manganese, silicon, sulfur, boron and numerous other lesser-known minerals are involved in bone synthesis, breakdown and repair. Given that the average North American diet has been shown to be deficient in these and other vital nutrients, it is easy to see why mineral deficiencies are part of the reason for the increasing incidence of osteoarthritis and other degenerative diseases.

Food allergies may be a hidden or unsuspected cause of chronic inflammation in a joint, leading to different types of arthritis including osteoarthritis. Some sufferers are sensitive to nightshade foods (tomato, potato, peppers, eggplant, tobacco) due to the presence of *solanine*, which may cause an inflammatory reaction in the joints. Sodium and iron supplements can also cause flare-ups in some sensitive individuals.

The Parasite Connection

There is a parasite connection to many common health problems experienced by both children and adults across North America. Parasites compete with us for nutrients like vitamins, minerals and amino acids and secrete waste products into our gut and bloodstream that are capable of causing various allergic and autoimmune reactions. While osteoarthritis is not necessarily caused by parasites, their presence in the body can certainly aggravate the signs and symptoms, making full recovery difficult.

If you have osteoarthritis and are not doing well with either conventional or natural treatments, visit a natural health care provider and get tested for parasites. While beyond the scope of this book, the treatment of parasites with diet, herbs, enzymes and even prescription drugs may be an important factor to consider as part of the treatment of resistant cases of osteoarthritis.

Conventional Treatments

Medical treatments do not address the cause of the disease and are aimed mainly at symptom relief. Simple painkillers like acetaminophen as well as anti-inflammatory drugs are used. Non-steroidal anti-inflammatory drugs (NSAIDS) do offer short-term pain relief, but they are not without side effects.

The US FDA reports 200,000 cases of gastrointestinal bleeding and up to 20,000 deaths yearly as a direct result of NSAIDS, kidney and liver damage.

NSAIDS may cause damage to the lining of the gastrointestinal tract and increase intestinal permeability, thereby increasing the number and severity of food allergies. A condition known as leaky gut syndrome may develop as a direct result of damage to the intestinal lining.

This breach in the gut wall allows invasion of the bloodstream by bacteria, fungi (candida) and parasites. The immune system then reacts to these foreign invaders as well as to tissues within the body that are similar in some way to the invaders. Most importantly, NSAIDS suppress cartilage repair. They are proven to worsen arthritis.

Therefore the aspirin, ibuprofen, indomethacin, piroxicam, diclofenac sodium and many others commonly prescribed for osteoarthritis, actually make it worse. And given that the integrity of the cartilage is of prime importance in preventing osteoarthritis, it is no wonder that the long-term use of such drugs have been proven to worsen arthritis.

On occasion, some doctors use injections of corticosteroids. These are anti-inflammatory hormones usually manufactured in the body in small amounts by the adrenal glands. Corticosteroids are secreted from the adrenals in higher amounts in response to illness and stress of any kind–they are the body's natural anti-inflammatory hormones.

Doctors who feel that osteoarthritis has become too severe to respond to NSAIDS or other painkillers often resort to injecting synthetic corticosteroids to completely suppress inflammation. Unfortunately, injected corticosteroids have many long-term side effects, not the least of which is osteoporosis.

Treating and Reversing Osteoarthritis . . . . .

It may take several decades for osteoarthritis to become severe enough to warrant medical attention, but the disease is reversible using a completely non-drug approach in six to twelve months on average. Better pain control can be achieved with a combination of diet changes and supplemental nutrients as early as six weeks after starting a natural treatment program. The following therapies are the ones that have worked best for my patients, or that have the best scientific support for their safety and efficacy.

Exercise and Physical Therapy

Exercise can be beneficial in treating osteoarthritis because strengthening ligaments, tendons and muscles will help stabilize a weakened joint. Physiotherapy, chiropractic, massage therapy and osteopathy can all be helpful in reducing the severity of the signs and symptoms of osteoarthritis.

Weight Loss

Maintaining one's ideal weight helps prevent osteoarthritis. Excess weight stresses all weight-bearing joints, including those in the spine, hips, knees, ankles and feet. A healthy weight-loss program using the eating guidelines discussed below will also help in reversing osteoarthritis.

Diet

The following recommendations are general guidelines only and should be modified depending on individual food tolerances or allergies. Nightshades foods (tomatoes, potatoes, peppers, eggplants, tobacco) might have to be eliminated by those who have joint pains associated with their consumption. There are certain foods (beef, pork and dairy, for example) that are proinflammatory: They increase the inflammatory response due to their content of certain types of fats (arachadonic acid and saturated fats) that increase the body's production of certain proinflammatory hormones called prostaglandins.

Non-steroidal anti-inflammatory drugs suppress cartilage repair and are proven to worsen arthritis.

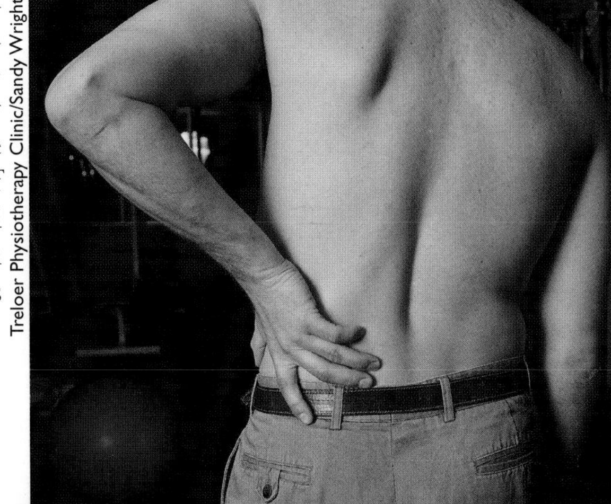

Treloar Physiotherapy Clinic/Sandy Wright

Other foods, like fish, flax and hempseed, are anti-inflammatory in that they have the reverse effect. Moreover, the foods in the prohibited category are the most allergenic and therefore the most likely to aggravate the inflammatory response. If you are not sure what foods or substances you might be allergic to, see a natural health care provider. You will find the menu suggestions and recipes that are included in this book helpful in planning your dietary transition.

Allowed Foods and Beverages

(provided you are not allergic to them)

- Carotene-containing foods like sweet potatoes, carrots, spinach, cantaloupe, kale, squash and pumpkin
- Rice cakes, rice cereals and rice crackers
- Vitamin C and antioxidant-containing foods such as citrus fruits, broccoli, strawberries, melons, Brussels sprouts and cabbages
- Popcorn (no butter or salt added)
- Buckwheat, quinoa, corn or rice pasta
- All fresh and dried fruits, preferably organic
- Lamb, poultry, fish and seafood, preferably organic (they must be well cooked)
- Organic fruit juices (freshly juiced if possible)
- Soy, rice or almond milk
- Small amounts of nuts (except peanuts and cashews)
- Sunflower and pumpkin seeds
- Pure, filtered or ozonated water (It is important for adults to drink at least eight large glasses each day.)

Foods to Avoid

- Wheat and other gluten-containing grains (barley, oats, rye, spelt, amaranth, millet and kamut)
- Milk and dairy products
- Eggs
- Sugar
- Artificial sweeteners (Stevia is a good non-sugar sweetener.)
- All alcoholic beverages, including beer and wine
- Caffeine (coffee, regular tea, colas, chocolate)
- Soft drinks and tap water (unless filtered by reverse osmosis or ozonated)
- All foods containing artificial flavorings, additives and preservatives
- Beef, pork, cold cuts, fried foods and salty foods
- Coconut
- Peanuts, cashews and their products

Food Allergy and Lab Tests

It has been known for eons that water or juice fasting for periods of several weeks may greatly improve or reverse arthritis. In fact, health spas that advocate fasting as a cure for arthritis achieve excellent results in reversing the disease. Research indicates that a fast reduces or eliminates the levels of circulating antibodies and the antigen-antibody complexes, which is extremely beneficial for arthritis sufferers.

Antibodies are made by our immune system in response to an antigen–a substance that is perceived by the immune system as an invader needing to be neutralized. An antigen-antibody complex is formed, and this elicits an inflammatory response. While this may be very useful in the case of invading viruses or bacteria, it can have a detrimental effect if the immune response is elicited by innocuous things like certain foods.

When the immune system starts to react in an aggressive way to harmless foods or its own organs, the antigen-antibody reaction could lead to a chronic inflammatory state each and every time an individual consumes an "allergic" food. Knowing what foods to eliminate reduces inflammation and subsequent arthritis.

All types of arthritis can be helped to varying degrees by detecting and eliminating food allergies. While the allergies themselves are not the cause of the arthritis, they may contribute to increasing the inflammatory response, making the signs and symptoms worse. In many cases, the elimination of the offending

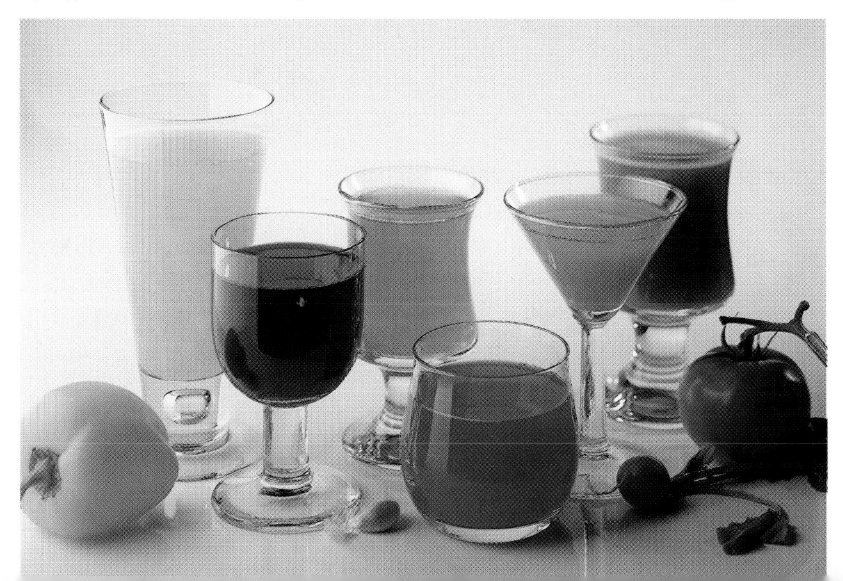

foods in itself may cause the arthritis to go into remission on a permanent basis.

To understand which types of tests are valid and reliable in determining food and chemical allergies, it is important to realize that there are basically only two kinds of adverse reactions: delayed and immediate. Unfortunately, this basic concept is still not firmly grasped by the majority of the population, nor by conventional allergists and pediatricians.

Allergic Reactions

The following is basic science fact:

Immediate (Type I) reactions:

- Allergic symptoms (e.g., wheezing, swelling, choking, pain) commonly occur two hours or less after consumption of the offending foods or chemicals. The food or chemical reaction is usually well known to the subject.
- There are only one or two foods involved in causing allergic signs and symptoms which are usually severe; for example, the well-known and often life-threatening reactions to peanuts, shellfish and strawberries.
- Food or chemical reactions are triggered by even trace amounts of foods. It may take only the odor of cooked lobster to elicit intense allergic reactions in sensitive individuals.
- Type I reactions are common in children and rare in adults.
- Reactions are usually a permanent or "fixed" allergy. These food reactions can be lessened by vitamin, mineral and herb supplementation.
- Associated with the IgE family of antibodies, Type I reactions can be verified by a skin test or a blood test called the IgE RAST (Radio-Allergo-Sorbent-Tests).

Delayed (Type II, III and IV) reactions

- Allergic reactions usually occur within twenty-four hours and sometimes up to four days after consumption of the offending foods or chemicals.
- There may be anywhere from three to twenty foods involved in causing allergic signs and symptoms, which are usually chronic (joint and muscle pain, fatigue, depression, psoriasis, etc.) and are hidden or unsuspected by the victim.
- Food or chemical reactions occur after consuming larger amounts of foods, often in multiple feedings. A single food challenge might not cause any allergic reactions to occur.
- These types of reactions are very common in children and adults; there are over fifty medical conditions and 200 symptoms triggered, worsened or caused by the allergic reactions.
- Reactions are usually reversible within three to six months with a combination of food elimination and nutritional supplement therapy (antioxidants, enzymes, herbs, etc.).
- These types of reactions can be verified by blood tests known as the ELISA/Act test, the non-IgE RAST and the FICA (Food Immune Complex Assay).

Most people with food allergies are unaware of their condition because in a delayed reaction the symptoms may occur many hours or days after ingestion. Delayed food allergies often create a complex blend of symptom-masking effects, withdrawal reactions and symptom reproduction with food reintroduction.

Those with food allergies can behave as if they were addicted to foods. People often crave the foods that cause their symptoms and this is one fairly reliable way of knowing what should be taken out of their diets to improve their immune status.

Since more than 90 percent of all food allergies are of the delayed onset type, skin tests and the IgE RAST will miss detecting the vast majority of food allergies. Nevertheless, conventional doctors continue to use them for that purpose, and often conclude that the patient does not have any food allergies even though no tests were ever done for delayed hypersensitivity food reactions. For this and other reasons, those suffering from arthritis, asthma, chronic sinusitis, hay fever, recurrent respiratory tract infections and other diseases are told that food allergies have nothing to do with their illness and that only a lifetime of steroid, antibiotic and antihistamine drugs will help.

There are many good tests that help detect food and chemical reactions. Although considerable confusion exists about which laboratory test is best, most agree with the accuracy and reliability of the elimination-provocation technique described by food allergy pioneers such as Drs. William Crook and Doris Rapp. This technique involves eliminating whole classes of foods for several days, then adding them back noting reactions.

Workable variations of this are the Coca Pulse Test and sublingual food tests. Some of these procedures would not be appropriate for those who do not have the time or stamina to experiment with their diets, or for people suffering from severe pain syndromes. On the other hand, there is something to be said for experiencing the effects of allergenic foods in reproducing symptoms. The elimination-provocation technique ultimately empowers sufferers to control symptoms with simple diet changes.

The Elimination-Provocation Test - The basic concept behind this type of food allergy testing is to follow a hypoallergenic diet for three weeks, eliminating the most common food allergens and thereafter challenging the body with the eliminated foods one by one, noting the reactions. During the three-week elimination diet, symptoms improve in the majority of people who suffer from food allergies. If the reintroduction of certain foods causes a reproduction of the symptoms, the person is probably allergic to those foods.

This diet works only if all the foods to be discontinued are done so abruptly or "cold turkey." Easing into this diet slowly or with some other compromise does not work nearly as well. In severely ill people (cancer, heart disease, diabetics, cortisone-dependent asthmatics or other life-threatening problems), this approach should be supervised by a medical doctor. Use common sense and the advice of your naturopath or doctor before attempting this on your own.

The elimination-provocation test (when appropriate) combined with the ELISA/Act test is currently state-of-the-art in detecting hidden food allergies. The scientific literature certainly supports this approach. The advantage of the ELISA/Act test is that it is capable of detecting delayed food allergies belonging to all of the delayed reaction.

This in no way invalidates other forms of testing that may work equally well for selected people. In the future, with more research, time and practitioner experience, the question of test validity and reliability will become clearer. In the meantime, people who eliminate the offending foods from their diets reduce the allergic load on the immune system. This gives the body the opportunity to repair damaged tissues like the joints, muscles or the lining of the respiratory tract.

Those who are allergic to dust, ragweed, pollens and other inhalant allergies can then be more tolerant to environmental allergens and less likely to suffer from severe allergic reactions that previously needed strong drugs for control.

Supplements

While the vast majority of people who change their diet as directed above experience improvement in their condition, osteoarthritis reversal can be accelerated or further enhanced with the use of a few natural remedies. Most of these compounds have been shown to be at least as effective as nonsteroidal anti-

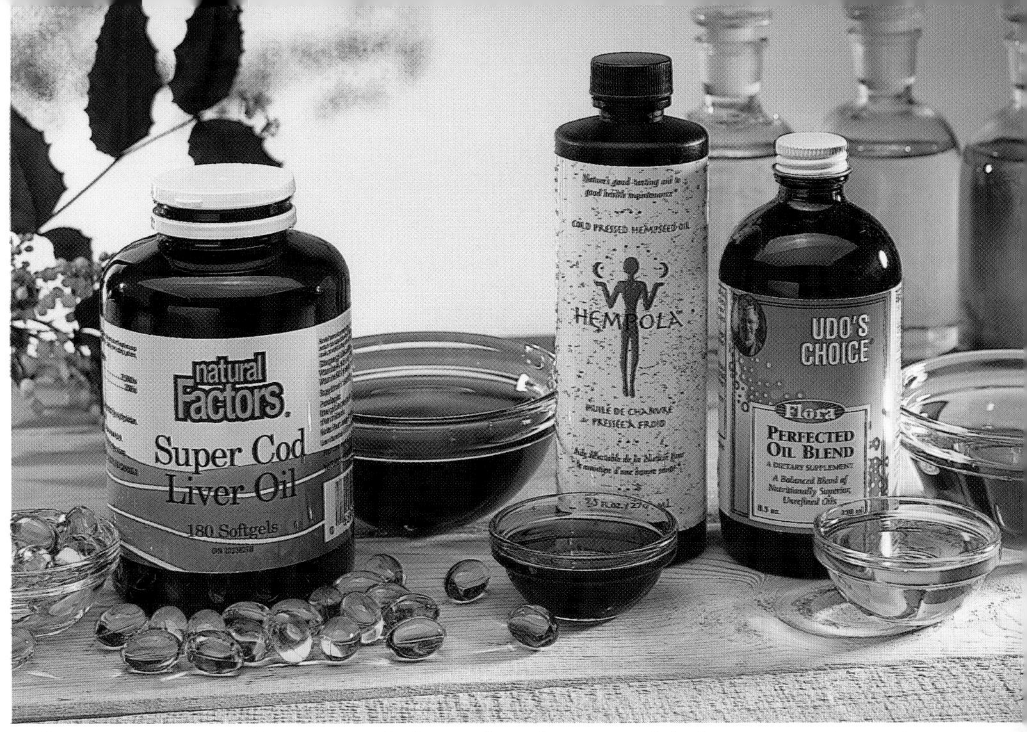

inflammatory drugs (aspirin and ibuprofen, for example) for controlling or eliminating symptoms. Some, like glucosamine sulfate, niacinamide and essential fatty acids, may be the keys to reversing the disease.

Essential fatty acids, along with glucosamine sulfate and niacinamide, may be the keys to reversing osteoathrithis.

For some people, cod liver oil will be enough to do the trick, while others may need to use a combination of six or more supplements for optimal symptom control. We are all biochemically unique, and consequently no single regimen will work equally well for one and all.

The following is a list of natural remedies that will help make diet and lifestyle changes work even better. Consult with your health care practitioner, and then experiment until you find the combination that works best for you.

Recommended Supplements (in order of importance):

Omega-3 Fatty Acids - Long before supplements like glucosamine sulfate became household names for reversing osteoarthritis, millions of people found great relief from joint pain, stiffness and reduced range of motion with daily cod liver oil. Cod liver oil works. It continues to help reverse osteoarthritis naturally, and is, I believe, first-line therapy for any inflammatory condition.

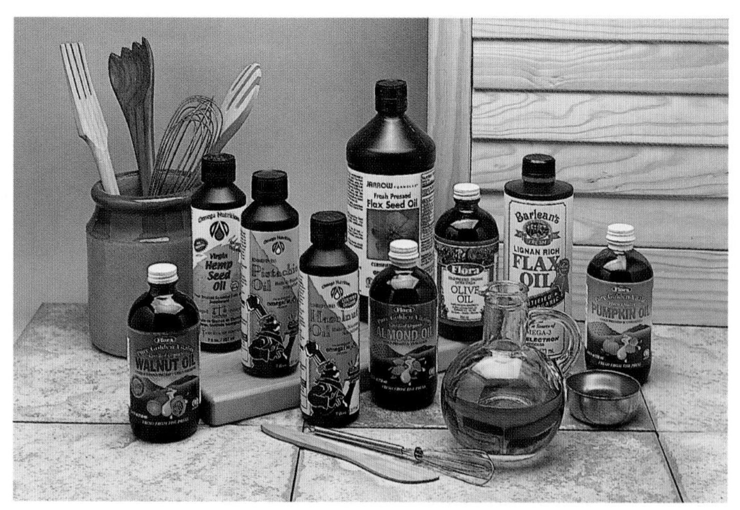

Cod liver oil, halibut liver oil and shark liver oil all contain fats that stimulate the body to manufacture anti-inflammatory hormones called prostaglandins. These fats, referred to as *eicosapentaenoic acid* (EPA), are found in large amounts in cold-water fish (trout, salmon, cod, halibut, mackerel, shark, etc.), and are highly effective as a natural anti-inflammatory agent. Good results can be anticipated in three to six months.

When combined with niacinamide and glucosamine sulfate, osteoarthritis can be significantly improved within six weeks or less.

Dosage: Typical therapeutic dosages are 9 to 12 grams daily of capsules, or two to three tablespoons of the oil.

Hempseed oil - Another more palatable source of essential fatty acids is hempseed oil, the production of which has recently been legalized in Canada. This oil contains nearly double the amount of anti-inflammatory essential fatty acids as other oils. It, too, is highly effective as an anti-inflammatory supplement.

Dosage: A typical dose is 2 to 3 tablespoons daily, taken straight or mixed with soups, salads or nut butters, such as almond or sesame.

Niacinamide - This B vitamin (a synthetic form of niacin) may enhance glucocorticoid secretion, a naturally produced anti-inflammatory adrenal hormone. If taking niacinamide, other B-complex vitamins should also be supplemented so as to achieve a proper balance of the complex. In one clinical study on the use of niacinamide (Vitamin B_3) seventy-two patients with osteoarthritis received either niacinamide or a placebo. Arthritis improved 29 percent in those taking niacinamide and worsened by 10 percent in the placebo subjects.

Niacinamide may help provide energy and nucleic acids to the cartilage itself, which may increase cartilage repair rates and complement the anti-inflammatory effect of other natural remedies. Treatment seems to be most effective when taken in frequent, divided doses (e.g., 500 milligrams six times daily rather than 1,000 milligrams three times daily).

Generally regarded as safe and effective without significant side effects, niacinamide in high doses can, nevertheless, cause nausea and liver irritation in the rare individual. If you have a history of liver disease, consult a physician before taking high doses of any nutritional supplement.

The beneficial effects of niacinamide begin to take effect between one and three months. Maximum benefits can be reached in one to three years.

Dosage: Suggested dosage is 500 milligrams six times daily.

Glucosamine sulfate - Numerous double-blind studies done in the 1980s concluded that supplementation with glucosamine sulfate reverses osteoarthritis. Other studies show it to be superior in pain relief to NSAIDS as it improves joint function and helps reduce the pain of those suffering from osteoarthritis.

Gucosamine sulfate actually works to repair the damage done by osteoarthritis, not just treat the symptoms. Its effectiveness in treating the damage results in effective pain relief as well. Double-blind studies show that glucosamine sulfate helps symptoms such as joint tenderness, pain on standing, pain on walking and joint swelling.

Gucosamine sulfate actually works to repair the damage done by osteoarthritis, not just treat the symptoms.

Glucosamine sultate is found in chitin, which is a portion of the exoskeleton found in yeasts, fungi and shellfish. Glucosamine helps bind water in the cartilage matrix and has been shown to help produce more collagen. It normalizes cartilage metabolism, the substance that helps to keep the cartilage from breaking down.

> "There is such a treatment that inhibits the degradation and actually starts rebuilding the cartilage, costs less, does not require a prescription, does not make the osteoarthritis worse by further destroying the cartilage, and does not have all of the extremely dangerous side effects of NSAIDS. This substance is glucosamine sulfate." - Sherry A. Rogers, MD, Health Counselor magazine

Glucosamine supplementation has produced a 95 percent response rate in patients compared to 72 percent in patients taking nonsteroidal anti-inflammatory drugs. It has been the drug of choice for treatment of osteoarthritis in Portugal, Spain and Italy since the early 1980s.

Do not confuse glucosamine sulfate with glucosamine hydrochloride. Many scientists believe that the sulfur component of glucosamine sulfate has a very important role to play, which cannot be replaced by hydrochloride. And all of the research on glucosamine was done with the sulfate form, not the hydrochloride. Be patient after deciding to take glucosamine sulfate.

Glucosamine supplementation has produced a 95 percent response rate from patients in pain relief compared to 72 percent from patients taking NSAIDS.

Remember that this supplement works naturally, re-building damage that has been done for long term relief and mobility. This work does not happen overnight. Do not expect to feel a significant difference before at least two months and be sure to take your dosage faithfully.

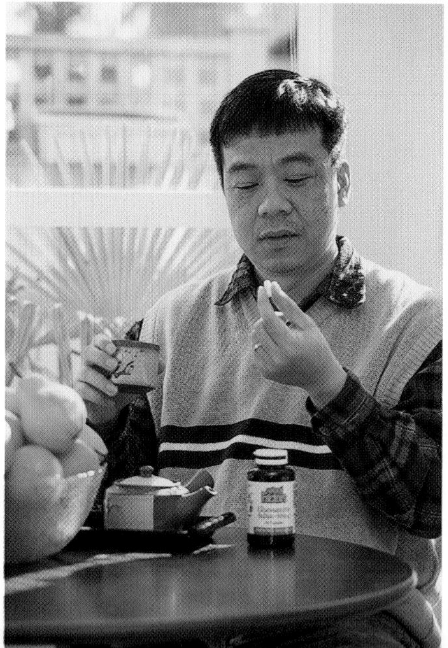

Glucosamine sulfate appears to be safe for just about anyone with osteoarthritis. Diabetics can take it without concern, since it does not raise blood sugar levels. While there are no significant side effects reported, some people with sensitive stomachs can feel a burning sensation if they take this supplement on an empty stomach. Taking glucosamine sulfate with meals can prevent stomach upset. If you have an ulcer, glucosamine sulfate should be used with caution. Using DGL (deglycyrrhizinated licorice) lozenges can be very soothing for ulcers and can be taken in combination with glucosamine sulfate. The usual way of using these is to chew, dissolve and swallow one or two DGL lozenges four times daily between meals for at least six weeks.

Dosage: The usual effective dose for adults is 500 milligrams three times daily.

Q and A on Glucosamine Sulfate (GLS)

Why don't doctors know about it?

By now, most doctors have heard of GLS and are prescribing it for their patients. Other physicians, set in their ways of practice, may be reluctant to prescribe natural remedies of any kind for fear of peer pressure or other professional chastisements. If your doctor has never heard of it, show him or her this book. Let your doctor know that the medical literature contains several dozen good studies supporting the use of GLS.

Why didn't my doctor tell me about it?

Most doctors are more comfortable prescribing drugs as opposed to something more natural. This is primarily because their medical education didn't cover natural therapies, only the drug and surgery approaches.

Can people with an allergy to shell fish take it?

Yes, because pure GLS contains no animal extracts.

Can I still take my NSAIDS?

Yes, but they are not likely to be necessary after two months of GLS combined with the arthritis diet and other natural remedies. NSAIDS should never be taken for indefinite periods of time due to their gastric hemorrhage potential. Make sure you take NSAIDS with food to prevent potential gastrointestinal problems.

How long will it take before I notice a difference?

GLS will work as effectively as NSAIDS within two months of starting the remedy in most people.

Shark and other cartilage products - Several studies indicate that supplementation of the diet with various preparations derived from animal tissues rich in glycosaminoglycans are successful treatments for osteoarthritis. The most popular of these is shark cartilage, perhaps better known for its ability to prevent the spread of cancer.

Other cartilage products from the lungs, trachea and bone marrow of cows and chickens have also been used with good results in arthritis. While these products are effective osteoarthritis remedies, their cost may be considerably higher than glucosamine sulfate, which appears to work as well or better than the animal extracts.

New Zealand Green-lipped mussel (Perna canaliculus) - This seafood is a rich source of glycosaminoglycans and eicosatetraenoic acids (ETAs), which are thought to be responsible for its beneficial effects in osteoarthritis and rheumatoid arthritis. The ETAs are potent inhibitors of leukotrienes, which are chemical mediators formed in the body that initiate and prolong the process of inflammation.

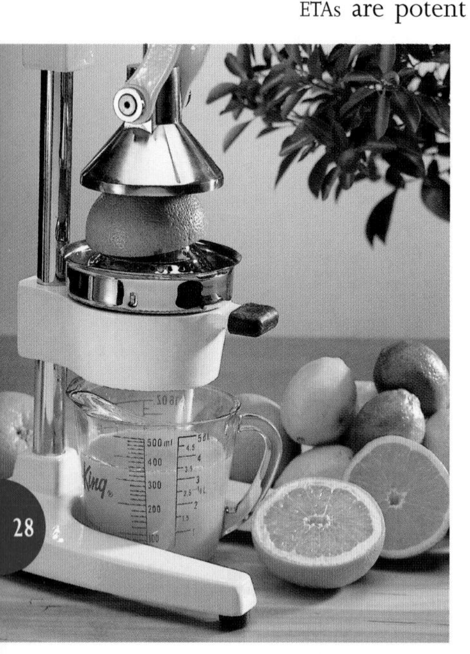

Vitamin C - High doses of vitamin C have been proven to have an anti-inflammatory effect in osteoarthritis. In one study involving 640 participants, high doses of vitamin C reduced the progression of osteoarthritis by a factor of three. This related mostly to a reduced risk of cartilage loss.

Those with high vitamin C intake also had a reduced risk of developing knee pain. A high intake of antioxidant nutrients, particularly vitamin C, may reduce the risk of cartilage loss and disease progression in people with osteoarthritis.

Dosage: Suggested dosage is 6,000 milligrams or more daily to bowel tolerance (the point at which diarrhea from the vitamin C occurs).

Vitamin E - At dosages of 800 IU daily, vitamin E may be a prostaglandin inhibitor similar to NSAIDS, but without the side effects. Vitamin E decreases the blood levels of lipid peroxides and has been proven to be superior to placebo with respect to pain relief.

One way in which vitamin E is thought to exert its anti-inflammatory effects is by stabilizing the lysosomal membranes found in all cells. If these membranes are disrupted, intracellular enzymes that cause joint damage could be released. Vitamin E helps prevent this from happening and thereby reduces the possibility of further joint destruction.

In at least two double-blind studies, vitamin E was shown to be significantly more effective than placebo in terms of pain relief and equally effective as one of the most frequently prescribed NSAID (diclofenac).

Dosage: 800 IU daily.

Vitamin D - Vitamin D plays an essential role in calcium metabolism; thus, daily intake of vitamin D from cod or halibut liver oil is an effective osteoarthritis treatment. This is one vitamin that can also be obtained in adequate amounts from exposure to sunshine: After twenty minutes in the sun a cholesterol derivative in the skin begins to manufacture vitamin D.

Dosage: 2,000 IU daily.

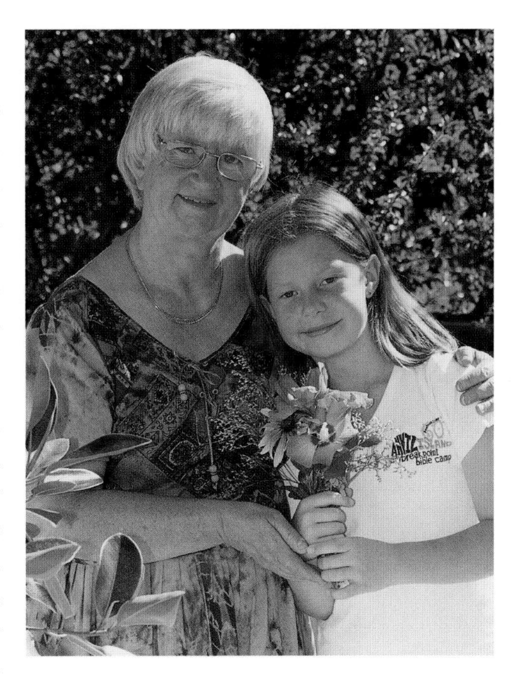

Adequate amounts of vitamin D can be obtained from exposure to sunshine.

Boron - Boron is essential to the body's synthesis of steroid hormones and vitamin D, both of which are vital for normal bone growth and repair. The dietary intake of the trace mineral boron may be inversely related to the risk of osteoarthritis. Boron is largely absent from the soils of countries where the incidence of osteoarthritis is high.

In parts of the world where boron intake is approximately 1 milligram or less daily, the incidence of osteoathritis in the population is between 20 to 70 percent. In areas of the world where routine boron intake is 3 to 10 milligrams per day, the estimated incidence of osteoarthritis is 0 to 10 percent.

Further, double-blind studies and clinical reports tell us that boron supplementation alone can reverse osteoarthritis in up to 90 percent of cases. The average adult under age seventy requires two months to improve signs and symptoms while those older than seventy need at least four months to see significant changes for the better. One can measure the amount of boron present in the body with a hair mineral analysis test.

While it is true that the potential for the body to make more estrogen and testosterone is enhanced with high dose boron supplementation, there is no evidence to suggest that using boron for extended periods of time increases the risk of any illness related to hormone intake. Clinical observations show boron is effective for 90 percent of arthritis patients.

Dosage: An effective dosage is 6 to 9 milligrams daily.

Selenium - Daily supplementation with selenium helps elevate levels of glutathione peroxidase, a selenium-containing antioxidant enzyme that is a potent free radical scavenger, which helps to reduce inflammation, pain and joint destruction.

Dosage: 200 to 600 micrograms daily.

Zinc and copper - Levels of these minerals are often low in those suffering from osteoarthritis. Hair mineral analysis is one way of assessing zinc and copper levels in the body. Copper bracelets have been used effectively for pain control for many years.

Dosage: Varies with individuals; consult with a health care practitioner.

Manganese - Manganese is an important component of articular cartilage, and is, therefore, helpful in treating osteoarthritis. Manganese is one of the most common mineral deficiencies due in part to the low levels of manganese in North American soil. It is conceivable that osteoarthritis symptoms will worsen owing to this dietary deficiency.

Like iron, calcium, zinc and copper, manganese requires proper amounts of stomach acid for its absorption. It may be deficient in people with a low output of stomach hydrochloric acid.

Dosage: 15 to 30 milligrams daily. Note: The best way of assessing for the levels of various trace minerals (manganese, zinc, copper, selenium) in the body is hair mineral analysis combined with blood tests to assess white cell or red cell levels of the same minerals.

It is also interesting to note that healthy levels of zinc, copper and manganese are needed by the body to manufacture superoxide dismutase (SOD), an enzyme which acts as a powerful free radical scavenger, reducing inflammation, pain and joint destruction occurring in osteoarthrtitis. Some studies have reported that injections of SOD will reverse osteoarthritis but oral SOD may not be well enough absorbed to accomplish the needed anti-inflammatory effects.

Zinc, copper and manganese supplementation, on the other hand, can increase the body's production of SOD and thereby reduce the signs and symptoms of osteoarthritis.

Chondroitin sulfates - The healing effects of chondroitin sulfate were all studied with the injectable form. Although poorly absorbed from the gastrointestinal tract, chondroitin sulfate taken orally appears to have a beneficial effect. When taken together, glucosamine sulfate and chondroitin sulfates work synergistically to stimulate cartilage production and help control enzymes that destroy cartilage.

Dosage: 500 milligrams three times daily with food

Methyl Sulfonyl Methane (MSM) - This natural form of organic sulfur is a critical component of the amino acids methionine, cysteine and cystine, which are contained in the cellular proteins of all living organisms.

Sulfur is needed for the proteins of hair, nails and skin, as well as for glutathione, one of the body's most important antioxidants.

A deficiency of MSM can result in fatigue and an increased susceptibility to arthritis. Methyl sulfonyl methane is present in raw fruits, vegetables and some grains, but is commonly lost during cooking, food processing and storage.

Sulfur baths and injections are traditionally effective therapies for arthritis used in health spas around the world. Many studies done in the 1920s and 1930s support the use of sulfur in reversing osteoarthritis. Studies also indicate that sulfur is commonly more deficient in those suffering from osteoarthritis than in people with normal, healthy joints.

While many proponents of MSM acknowledge the effectiveness of glucosamine sulfate, they are also quick to say that it is the sulfur component of this popular arthritis remedy that produces all the beneficial results. Combining glucosamine sulfate with MSM may well make both treatments work better than either one taken alone.

Methyl sulfonyl methane is an odorless and stable metabolite of DMSO, which was a short-lived fad treatment for arthritis and other sports related injuries. When DMSO is applied to the skin, it is rapidly absorbed into the circulation and provides pain relief to the affected areas.

The drawback to DMSO therapy is that it gives users a powerful garlic odor, making its use unpopular to all but the most motivated. Methyl sulfonyl methane is as powerful in its effects as DMSO but there is no offensive odor.

Long used in veterinary medicine as a supplement to control arthritic pain, MSM also has proven therapeutic benefits in humans. Side effects and toxicity have not been reported. Aside from its benefits in osteoarthritis, MSM has been promoted as an effective remedy for gastrointestinal upsets, allergies, skin problems, parasitic infestations, cancer prevention and to boost the immune system.

Dosage: The standard adult dose of 6 to 12 grams daily is most effective when combined with vitamin C (3 to 6 grams daily).

Cetyl Myristoleate (CMO) - This supplement is another natural antiarthritic agent. Cetyl myristoleate is made by using the myristoleic acid from bovine sources. It is a modified fatty acid used to treat rheumatoid arthritis and other autoimmune diseases; it has also been shown to be significantly effective against osteoarthritis as well. Some studies have shown that it increases the effectiveness of glucosamine sulfate.

It seems to act as a lubricating agent to the joint. Despite claims to the opposite, there are no plant or vegetarian sources of CMO.

This supplement is fairly expensive, and buyers should be aware that not all the available products on the market, especially those claiming a vegetarian source, are effective against arthritis. Success rate is 60 to 75 percent for arthritis pain relief. Side effects are rare to non-existent.

Dosage: Most health care professionals experienced with the use of CMO recommend it in the range of 12 to 15 grams per course of therapy. However, some people have reported significant improvement with as little as 3 to 4 grams. Do not take for extended periods of time or on a continued basis.

Cat's Claw (Uncaria tomentosa) - This herb comes from the Peruvian rainforest. Cat's claw has been proven to have pronounced anti-inflammatory and immune-stimulating properties. Health care providers are now using it successfully for osteoarthritis patients.

Dosage: 500 to 1,000 milligrams three times daily with food, or 1 teaspoon of tincture three times daily.

Devil's Claw (Harpagagophytum procumbens) - Devil's claw root is a South African plant observed to have an action comparable to that of phenylbutazone (an NSAID) in several European studies. Besides anti-inflammatory glycosides, devil's claw also contains numerous complex constituents including the phytosterols, B-sitosterol and stigmasterol, unsaturated fatty acids, triterpenes, and flavonoids. Its low toxicity potential makes it worth trying as part of a comprehensive natural regime to reverse osteoarthritis.

Dosage: 500 milligrams three times daily with meals.

Enzymes - Plant-based digestive enzymes (bromelain, papain) and pancreatin enzymes (animal based) are often used as oral supplements to enhance digestion. When these are taken on an empty stomach (about one hour before or after food), they enter the bloodstream and work as a powerful anti-inflammatory agent, reducing pain, swelling and infection while improving joint flexibility.

A recent study confirms that oral digestive enzyme supplements will work as well as prescription non-steroidal anti-inflammatory drugs in controlling the pain of osteoarthritis. A double-blind, randomized study (Clin Drug Invest 19(1):15-23, 2000) concludes that pain relief equivalent to that produced with prescription NSAIDS can be accomplished within three weeks of using over-the-counter proteolytic (breaks down undigested protein) digestive enzyme supplements containing bromelain, trypsin and rutin.

Adding a proteolytic digestive enzyme supplement containing bromelain, papain, trypsin, pancreatin and other enzymes has been reported to reverse inflammation in not only osteoarthritis but also tendinitis (e.g., tennis elbow), bursitis, vasculitis, nephritis and any other condition ending in -itis. If you have inflammation of any kind, consider using digestive enzymes on an empty stomach several times each day.

Dosage: Five capsules three times daily on an empty stomach.

Boswellia serrata - Boswellia is a herb native to India. It has well proven anti-arthritic effects through the inhibition of inflammatory medicators, prevention of decreased cartilage formation and improved blood supply to the joints. While it appears to be effective on its own, boswellia is often seen in combination products containing bromelain, yucca, devil's claw, glucosamine sulfate, curcumin or other natural compounds. No side effects have ever been reported with the use of boswellia.

Dosage: 400 milligrams three times daily.

Ginger (Zingiber officinale) - Regular supplementation for three months or longer can reduce pain, swelling an inflammation in osteoarthritis in 75 percent of people. Ginger is soothing for not only inflamed joints but also any inflamed parts of the gastrointestinal tract. It is also very well known and effective in the treatment of nausea, motion sickness or morning sickness in pregnancy. There are no known side effects.

Ginger

Dosage: 1,000 milligrams or more four times daily.

Yucca - A saponin extract of the desert yucca plant has been demonstrated to help reverse osteoarthritis within three months of use without side effects.

Dosage: 500 milligrams four times daily.

Velvet elk antler - Velvet elk antler has been used as a nutritional supplement in China for over 2,000 years. As important in traditional Chinese medicine as ginseng, velvet elk antler is said to prevent aging, boost energy and enhance immunity. It has started to become a popular supplement in Canada and the US owing to its antiarthritis effects.

Velvet elk antler is a renewable resource that is harvested humanely each year from specially bred elk during the rapid growth phase of antler development.

Dosage: 500 to 1,000 milligrams daily. Caution: Although no significant side effects have been reported with velvet elk antler, it is advisable to check with your doctor before self-administering, especially if you are currently being treated for a medical condition.

Oil of oregano - Oil of oregano has been used successfully as an anti-arthritis, anti-inflammatory remedy by millions. Compounds found in this supplement also act as free radical scavengers (shield against toxins), thus preventing further tissue damage while encouraging healing.

Dosage: Two or three drops (mixed with some olive oil to improve palatability) under the tongue several times daily, or applied topically.

S-Adenosylmethionine (SAM) - This supplement has been used extensively in Europe for the treatment of osteoarthritis. It has only recently become available in Canada and the US. This product is a metabolite of the essential amino acid methionine, which acts as a methyl donor in numerous biochemical reactions throughout the body. It stimulates the synthesis of proteoglycans, which provide essential nutrition for cartilage cells.

The only real problem with SAM is the cost: At present time, a bottle of twenty tablets costs approximately CND $30, making long-term usage of this remedy beyond the reach of most. If the price were something more in line with the inexpensive but very effective cod liver oil and niacinamide products, SAM would certainly be closer to the top of this list.

Dosage: 200 to 400 milligrams three times daily.

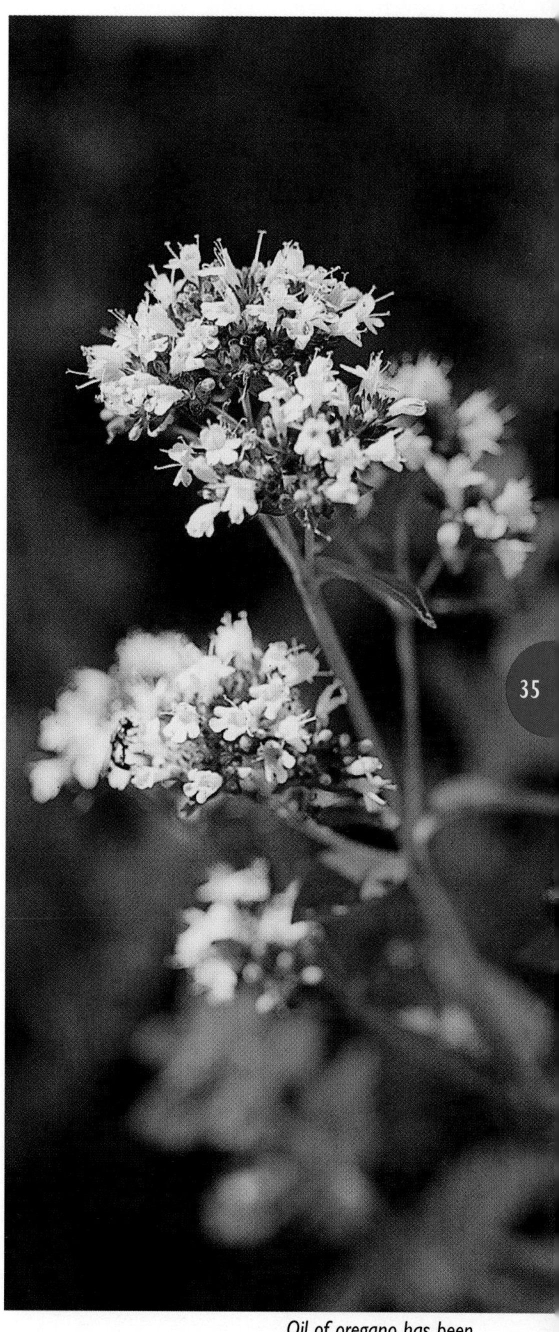

Oil of oregano has been successfully used by millions to treat arthritis.

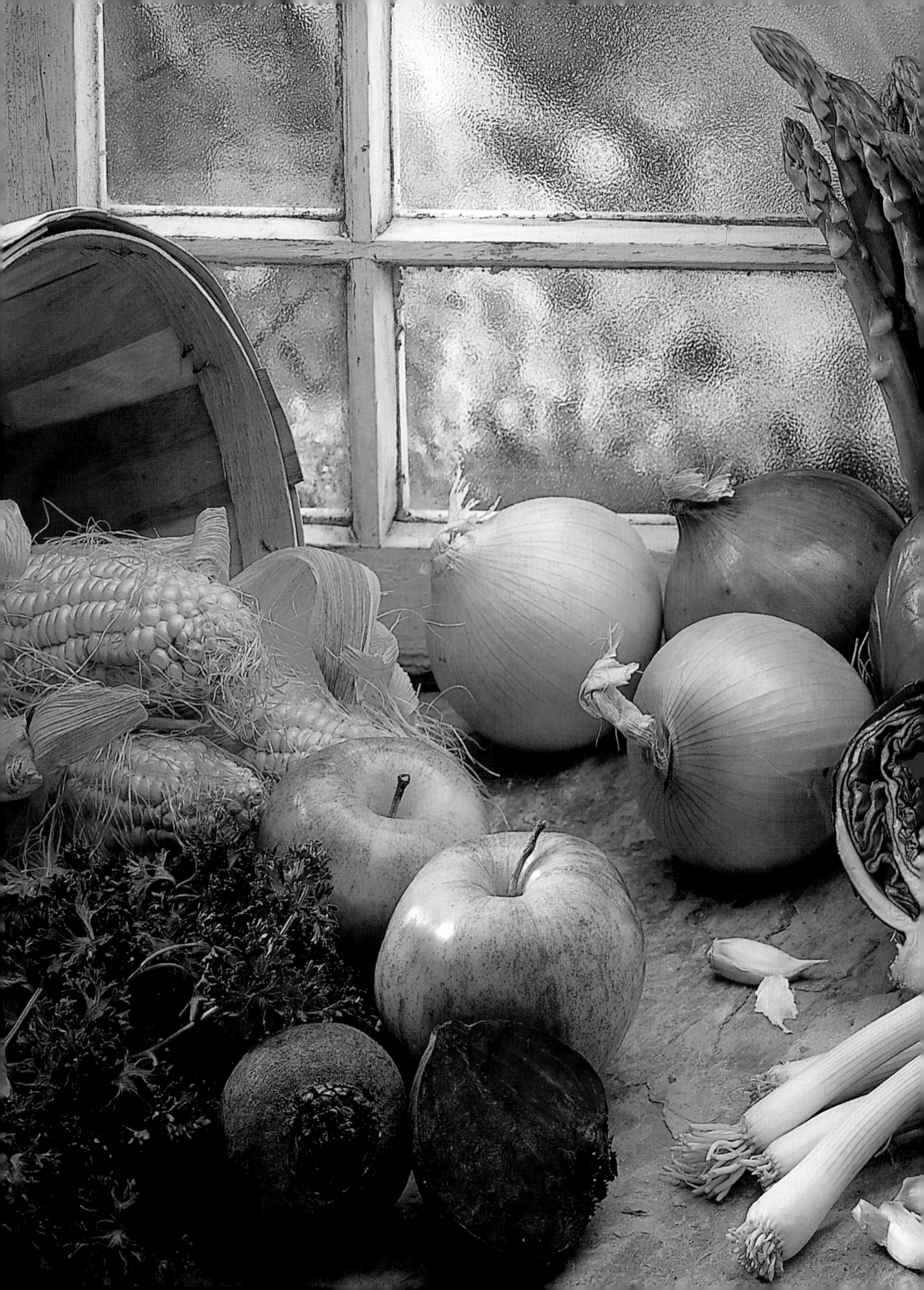

Healthy Recipes

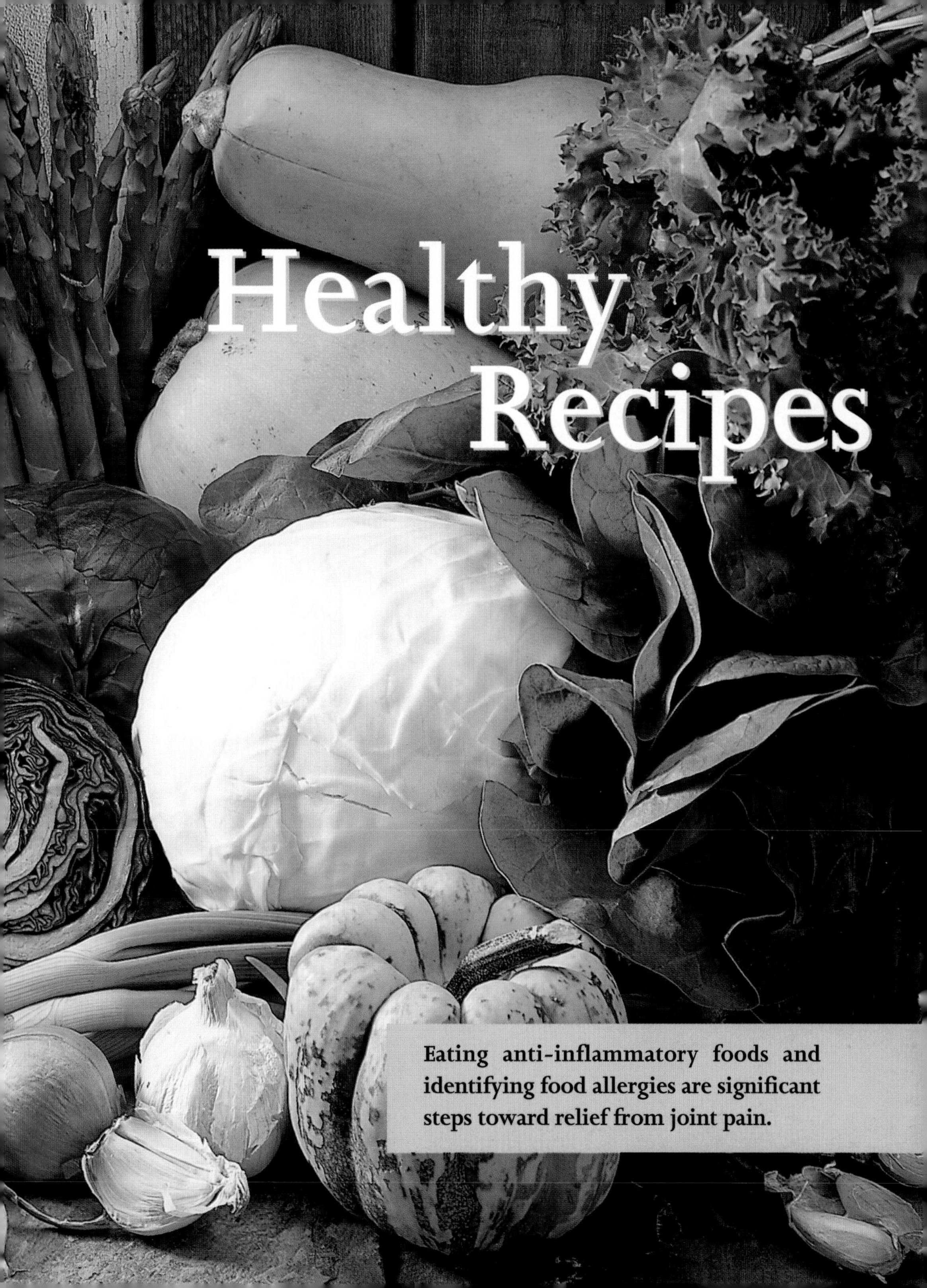

Eating anti-inflammatory foods and identifying food allergies are significant steps toward relief from joint pain.

Healthy Start Breakfast

Kiwis contain twice as much vitamin C as oranges so, with these two fruits combined, you'll start the day loaded with antioxidants.

2 medium ripe kiwis, peeled and sliced

1 large orange, peeled and segmented

1 organic Granny Smith apple, peeled and sliced

1 tbsp cold-pressed flax seed oil

1 tsp freshly squeezed lemon juice

1 bowl corn or quinoa flakes

1 cup (250 ml) **rice milk**

In a bowl, gently combine the fruit then drizzle oil and lemon juice over top. Add corn flakes and mix gently together. Pour rice milk over top and serve immediately.

Serves 1

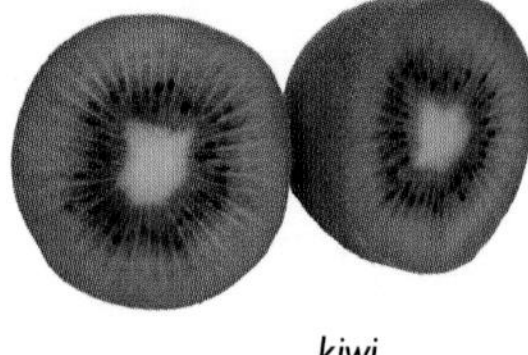

kiwi

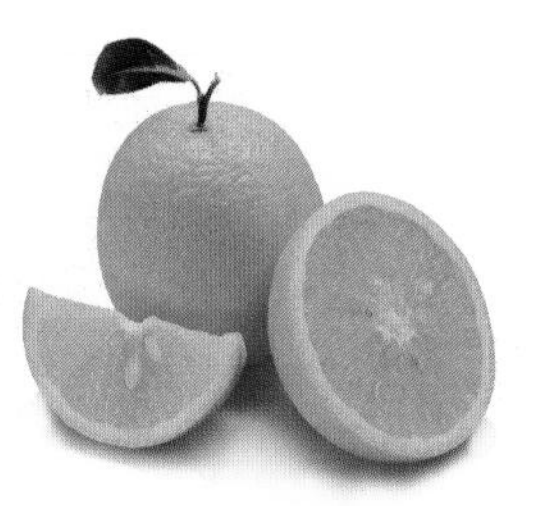

orange

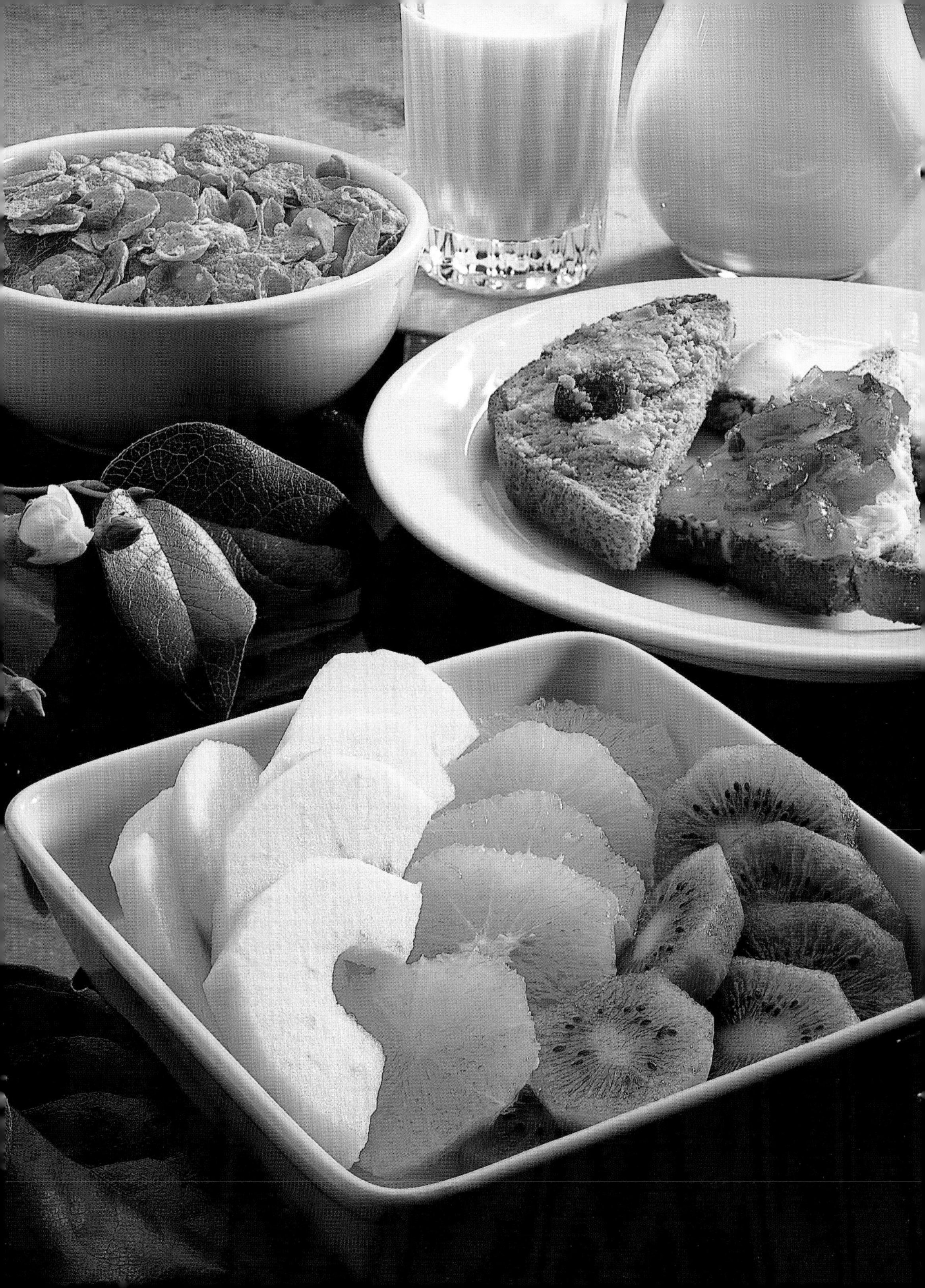

Pink Grapefruit and Avocado Salad

They say what's good for your heart is good for your health, because your heart is the engine that drives your body. Grapefruit is good for a healthy heart and is also known to lower the risk of cancer and lower blood cholesterol. The avocado in this salad will supply a high amount of the healthy fats your body needs to function properly. Together these foods equal not only a delicious salad, but a healthy meal.

2 pink grapefruits, peeled and segmented

2 ripe avocados, cut in 1" cubes

2 hearts butter lettuce

2 tsp fresh thyme, chopped

Sea salt to taste

Dressing:

½ cup (120 ml) cold-pressed flax seed oil

1 tbsp freshly squeezed lemon juice

1 tbsp maple syrup or honey

1 tsp sweet Dijon mustard

Wash and thoroughly dry lettuce leaves. Place the lettuce in the shape of cups in the center of serving plates. Mix the remaining ingredients, including the mixed dressing, and place in the center of the lettuce cups.

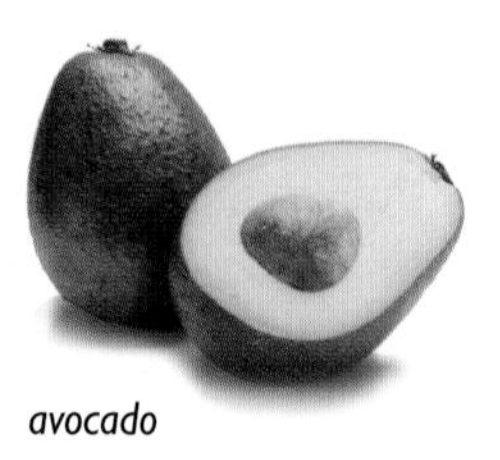

avocado

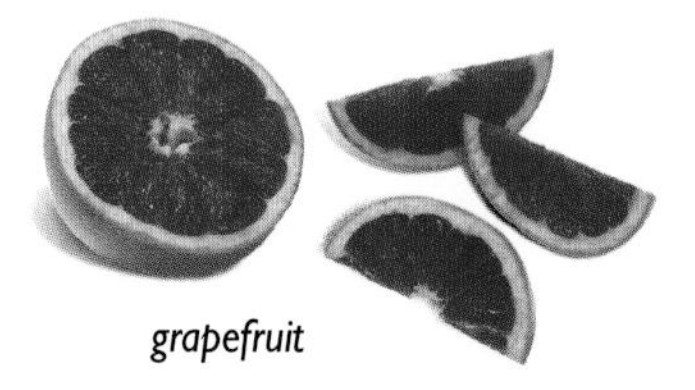

grapefruit

The white part of the grapefruit on the inside of the peel is called the "pith." Many of the nutrients of the fruit are located here. Squeeze the liquid from the pith into your dressing for added vitamins and minerals.

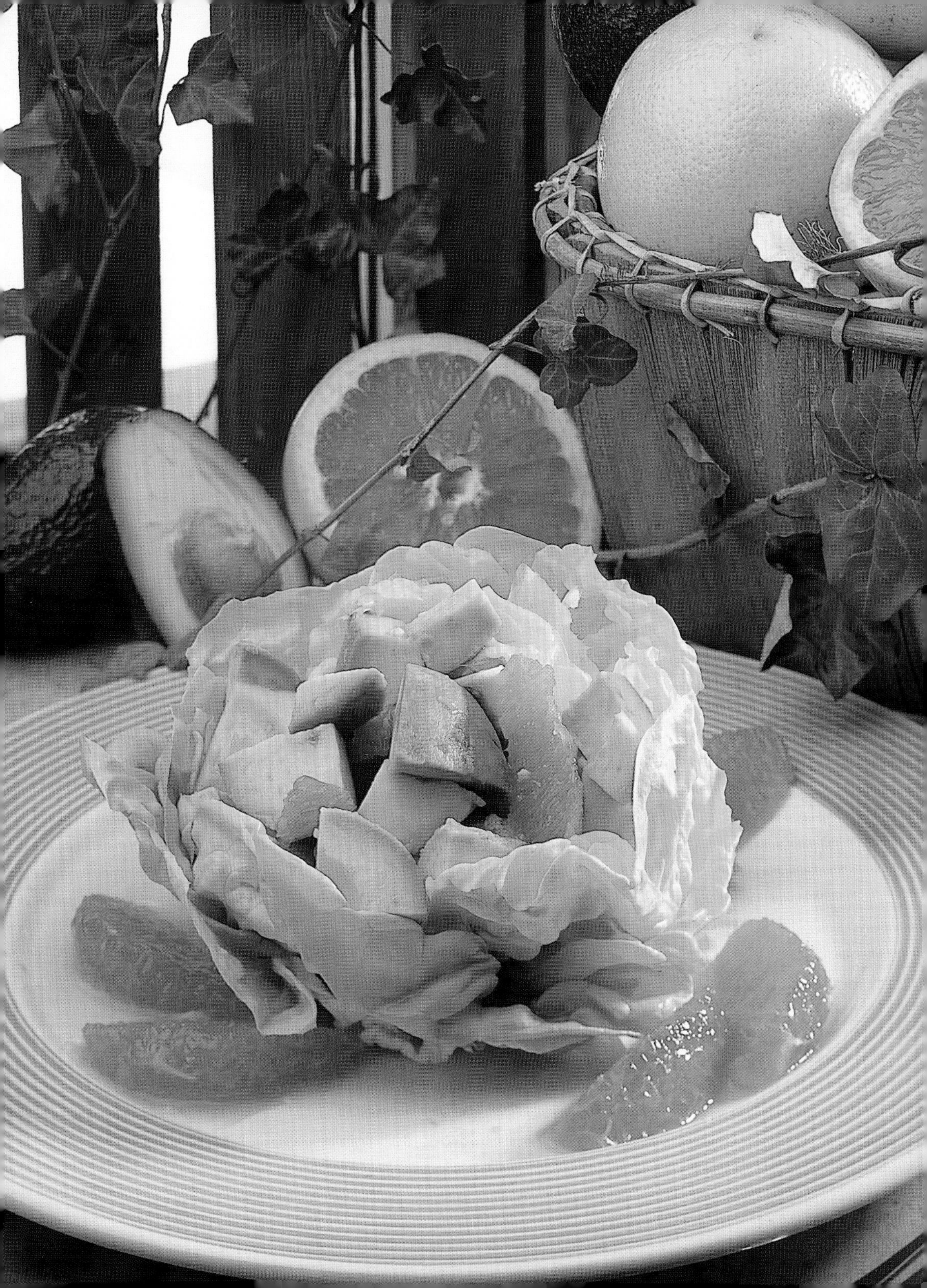

Baby Romaine with Tropical Fruit

Mangos used to be found only in the tropics, but they are now available year round and in every corner of the world. They provide an abundance of vitamins A and C and good amounts of potassium.

3 baby romaine hearts, leaves separated

1 large ripe mango

1 large firm papaya

¼ cup (80 g) sunflower seeds

Dressing:

2 tbsp cold-pressed walnut, flax seed or olive oil

1 tbsp freshly squeezed lemon juice

1 tbsp freshly squeezed orange juice

1 tbsp cold-pressed sunflower seed oil

Pinch curry powder

Sea salt, to taste

Peel mango and papaya, remove seeds and cut into 1" chunks.

In a large bowl, whisk together all the dressing ingredients. (Using a hand mixer will give more volume.) Add romaine, mango, papaya and sunflower oil and toss well. Serve immediately.

Serves 2

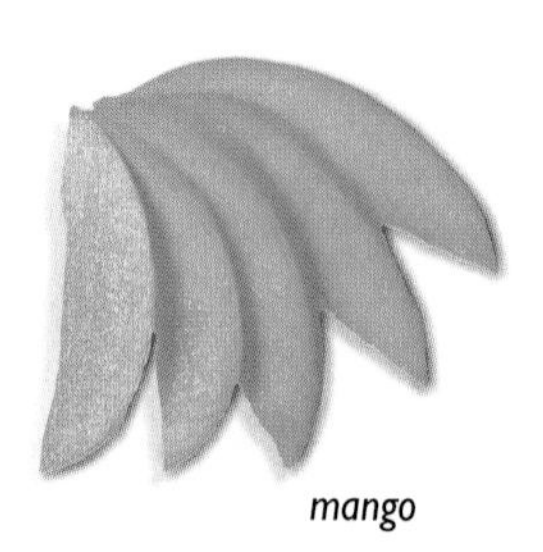

mango

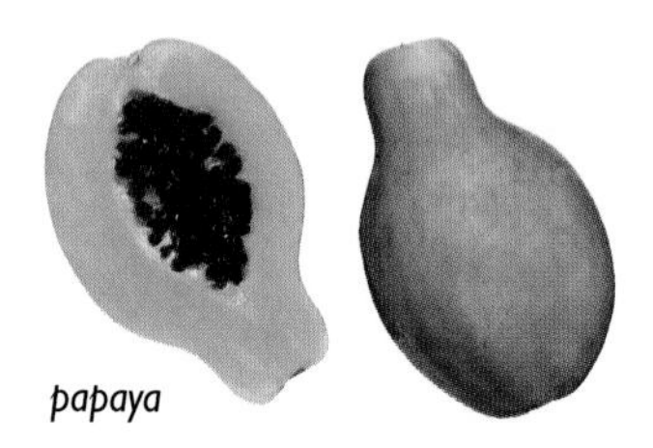

papaya

Baby romaine comes from the heart of the romaine lettuce and its leaves are sweet and tender. If you don't want to use the baby romaine, simply tear the large romaine leaves into smaller pieces.

A firm, slightly green, papaya contains more enzymes than a ripe one.

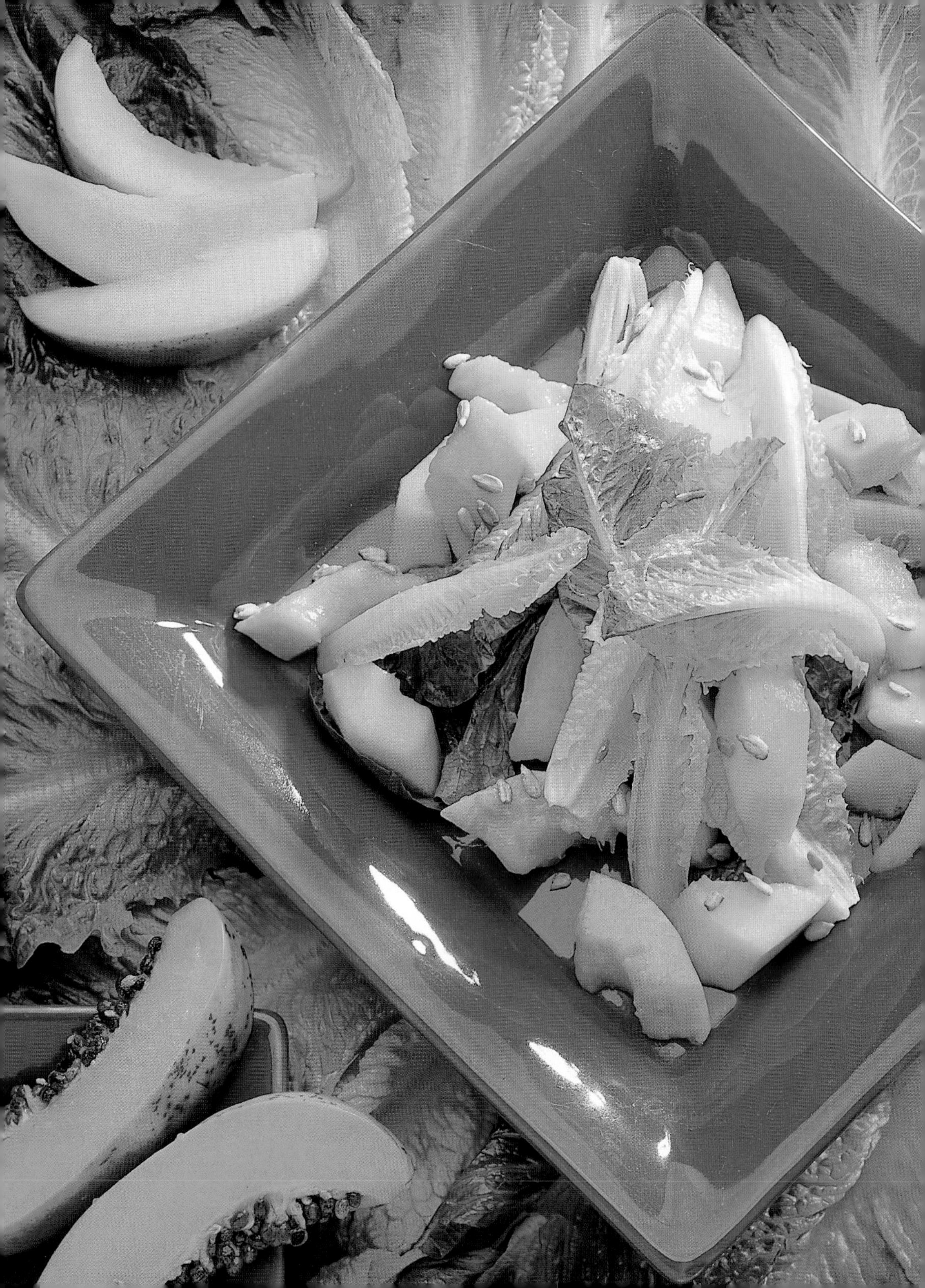

Watercress Salad with Lentils

Traditionally, lentils were a food for the poor-Catholic people who could not afford fish. Today, lentils are appreciated for their versatility and nutritional benefits. They contain an abundance of protein, vitamin A, and a variety of minerals, including calcium and magnesium.

½ cup (225 g) **red lentils**

4 Brussels sprouts, quartered

2 cups (300 g) **watercress**

1 cup (240 g) **grapes, sliced**

1 shallot, minced or 2 tbsp green onion, chopped

1 cup (150 g) **alfalfa sprouts**

Dressing:

2 tbsp extra-virgin olive oil

2 tbsp cold-pressed pumpkin seed oil

2 tbsp grape juice

1 tbsp freshly squeezed lemon juice

1 tbsp fresh mint, chopped

Bring a pot of water to a boil, add lentils and cook for 5 to 8 minutes. Add Brussels sprouts and cook for an additional 4 minutes. Drain and rinse well with cold water.

In a large bowl, whisk together all dressing ingredients. Add Brussels sprouts, lentils, watercress, grapes and shallot and toss well. Garnish with alfalfa sprouts and serve immediately.

Serves 2

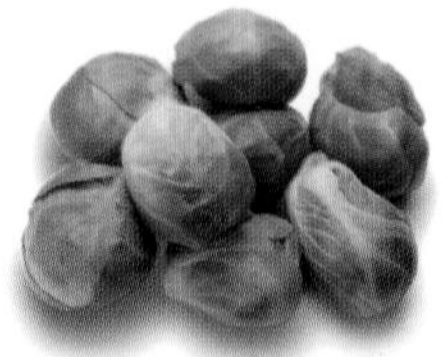

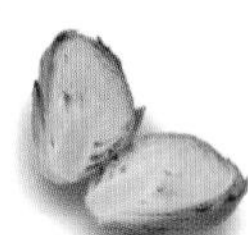

Brussels sprout

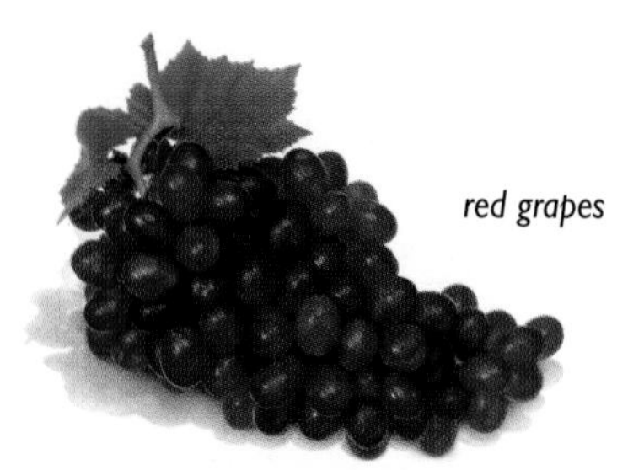

red grapes

Lentils do not need to be soaked overnight as they cook more quickly than other beans.

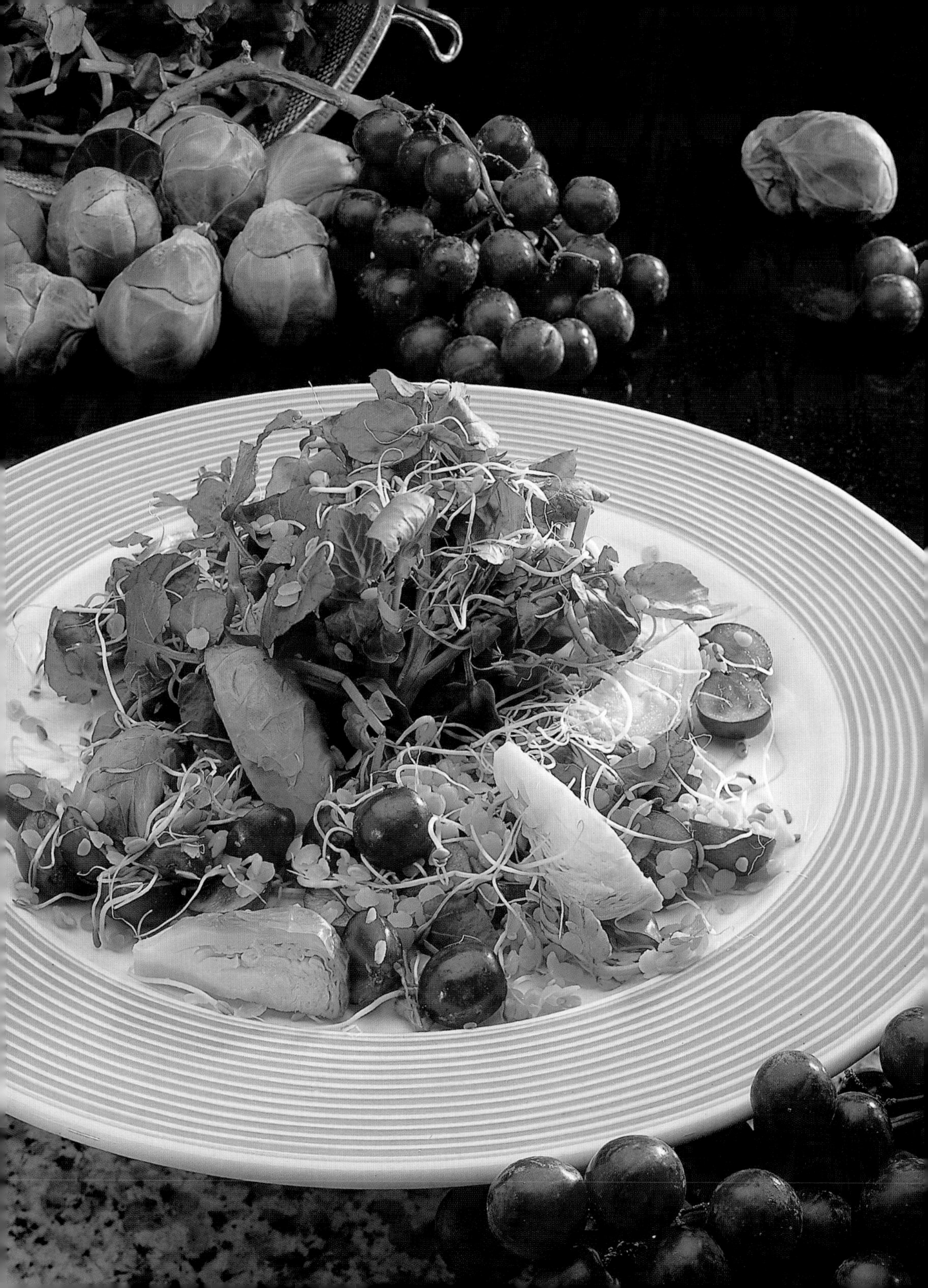

Corn and Avocado Soup

The avocado, which is actually a fruit, contains a fabulous amount of the good fats that our bodies need, along with a significant amount of protein and vitamin E. The essential fatty acids and protein stimulate tissue growth and healing. Corn is a bone and muscle builder and also provides a wealth of vitamins and minerals.

1 ripe avocado, thinly sliced

2 cups (450 g) **fresh or frozen corn kernels**

3 tbsp extra-virgin olive oil

1 cup (240 g) **celery, diced**

1 cup (240 g) **white onion, diced**

2 cloves garlic, minced

3 cups (750 ml) **vegetable stock or water**

Zest of 1 lemon

2 bay leaves

Pinch ground nutmeg

Sea salt to taste

1 tbsp fresh cilantro, chopped for garnish

In a large pan, heat oil over medium heat and sauté the celery, onion and garlic until tender. Add corn, sauté for an additional 2 minutes, then add the vegetable stock, lemon zest, bay leaves, cayenne and nutmeg. Cover and simmer for 5 to 7 minutes then remove from heat.

Remove the bay leaves. Place the mixture in a blender and blend until smooth. Season with salt and pepper. Pour the soup into bowls then place avocado slices over top. Garnish with cilantro and serve immediately.

Serves 2

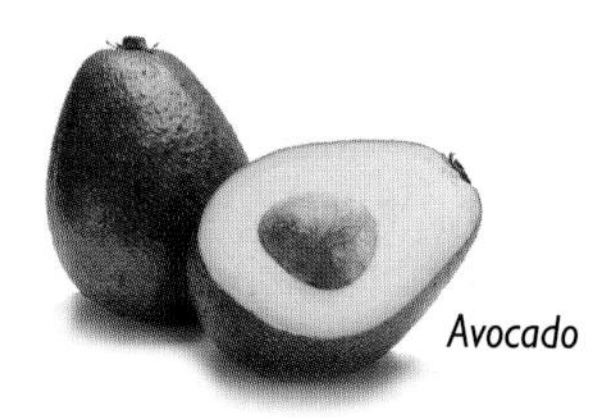

Avocado

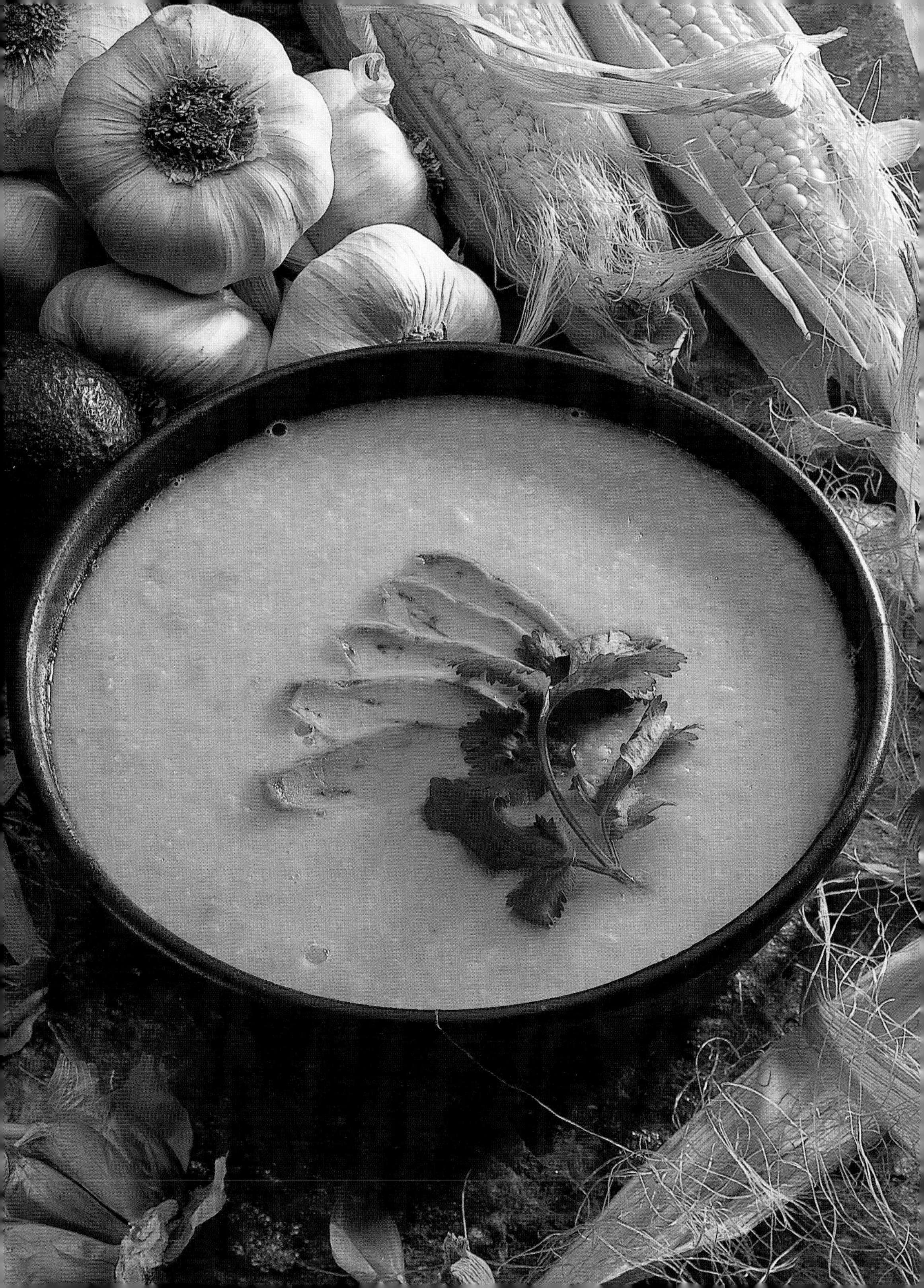

Green Pea Soup with Polenta Dumplings

Many of us have fond childhood memories of eating peas fresh from the pod, and so we'll always find room for a bowl of pea soup. Green peas are high in A and B-complex vitamins and are a good source of potassium and calcium. They also contain the same amount of soluble fiber as kidney beans.

Soup:

2 cups (450 g) **fresh or frozen green peas**

3 tbsp extra-virgin olive oil

1 cup (225 g) **white onion, diced**

2 cloves garlic, minced

1 cup (225 g) **celery, diced**

2 cups (450 ml) **vegetable stock or water**

1 bay leaf

Pinch ground nutmeg

Sea salt to taste

2 tbsp fresh parsley, chopped

Dumplings:

½ cup (125 g) **polenta** (coarse corn) **flour**

1 cup (250 ml) **water**

Pinch sea salt

¼ cup (60 g) **fresh corn kernels**

1 tbsp fresh thyme leaves

Sea salt to taste

1 tbsp extra-virgin olive oil

To prepare the soup, heat oil in a large pot over medium heat and sauté onion, garlic and celery until tender. Add peas, vegetable stock, bay leaf and nutmeg. Season with salt and pepper. Cover and simmer for 5 to 7 minutes. Remove the bay leaf.

Pour the soup into a food processor and purée it until smooth. Return to the pot, add parsley, stir and keep warm.

To make the polenta dumplings, bring the water and a pinch of salt to a boil in a medium-size pot. Slowly add polenta, stirring constantly with a wooden spoon for 7 to 10 minutes. Reduce heat to medium. Before the polenta starts to thicken, stir in corn and thyme, and season with salt and pepper. Add olive oil and stir until thick. Scoop up some dough using a teaspoon. With another teaspoon, form the dough into an oval shape by scraping the dough from one teaspoon to the other.

Pour the soup into bowls, add the dumplings and serve immediately.

Serves 2

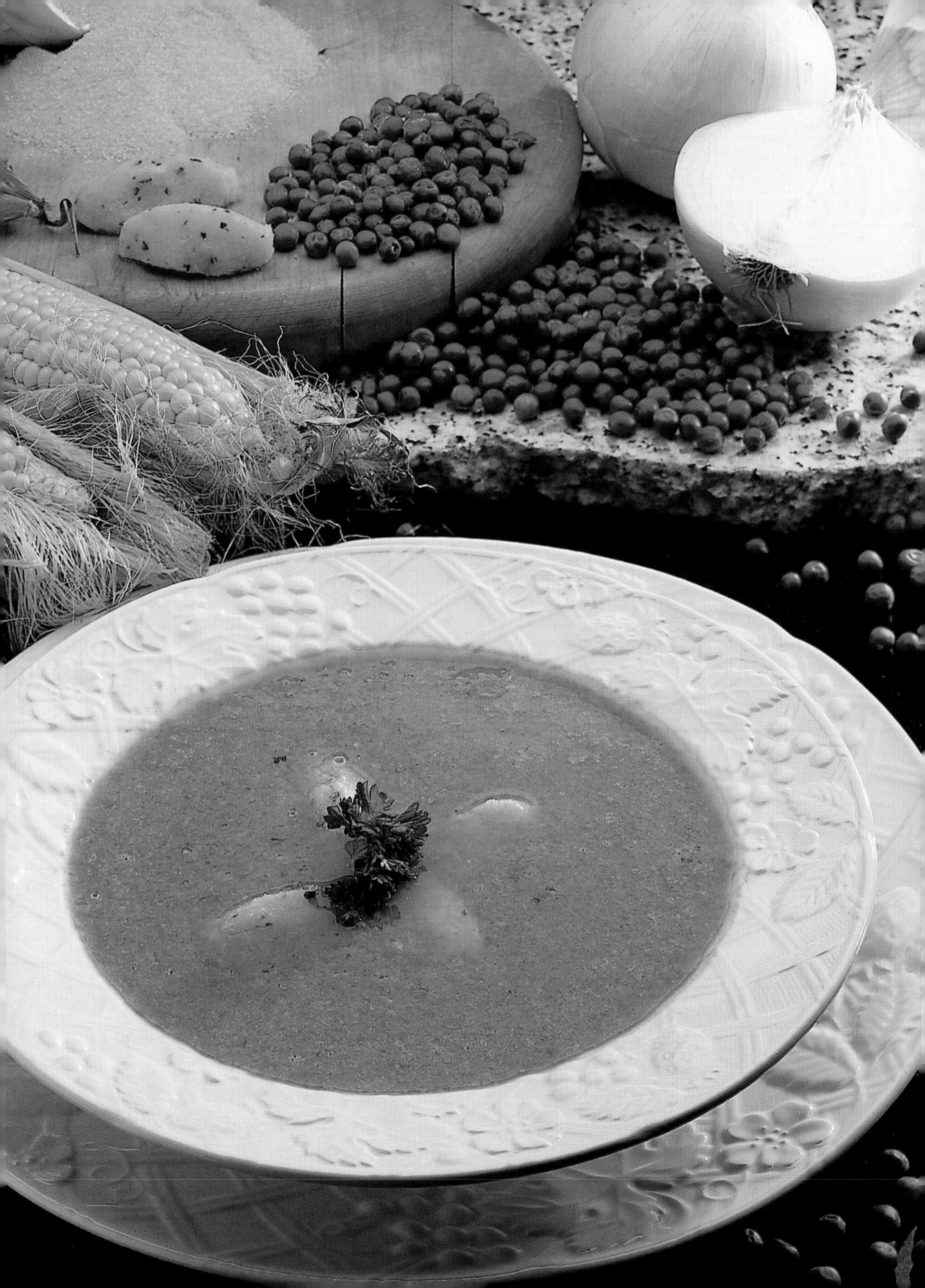

Ruben Sandwich with Roasted Yam

Cabbage is eaten worldwide and has long been a staple for frugal cooks. It is such a healthful food, almost all conditions, including osteoarthritis, can benefit from its therapeutic effects and immune-boosting properties. It is rich in vitamins A, C and K and contains good amounts of minerals.

- **2 large yams**
- **2 tbsp cold-pressed olive oil**
- **1 cup** (240 g) **white onion, sliced**
- **2 cups** (350 g) **white mushrooms, sliced**
- **3 cups** (450 g) **white cabbage, finely shredded**
- **1 tsp caraway seeds**
- **Sea salt to taste**
- **4 slices quinoa bread, toasted**
- **1 tbsp butter**
- **1 tbsp cold-pressed flax seed or pumpkin seed oil**
- **1 ½ cups** (150 g) **alfalfa sprouts**

Preheat the oven to 380°F (200°C).

To prepare the yams, wash them carefully with the skin on then cut them lengthwise in ½" (1 cm) wedges. Bring a pot of water to a boil, add the yams and cook them for 5 to 7 minutes or until slightly tender. Drain and rinse yams with cold water, then dry them thoroughly with a paper towel. Brush them with 1 tablespoon of olive oil and place in the oven for 10 to 12 minutes, turning once, until both sides are golden brown. Keep the yam warm in the oven.

In a frying pan, heat 1 tablespoon of olive oil over medium heat and sauté the onion, mushroom and cabbage until tender and slightly brown. Add caraway seeds and season with salt and pepper.

To assemble the sandwich, butter two slices of bread, place the cabbage mixture over top of each slice and drizzle with flax seed oil. Top with alfalfa sprouts and remaining bread. Serve with the roasted yams.

Serves 2

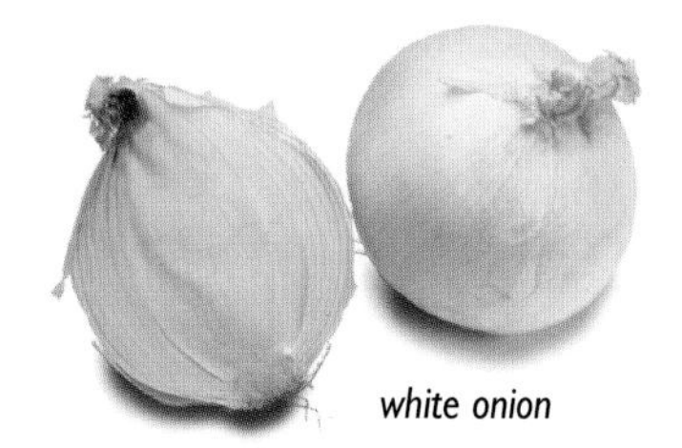

white onion

Fresh carotene- and antioxidant-rich fruits, such as cantaloupe and strawberries, go well with this dish.

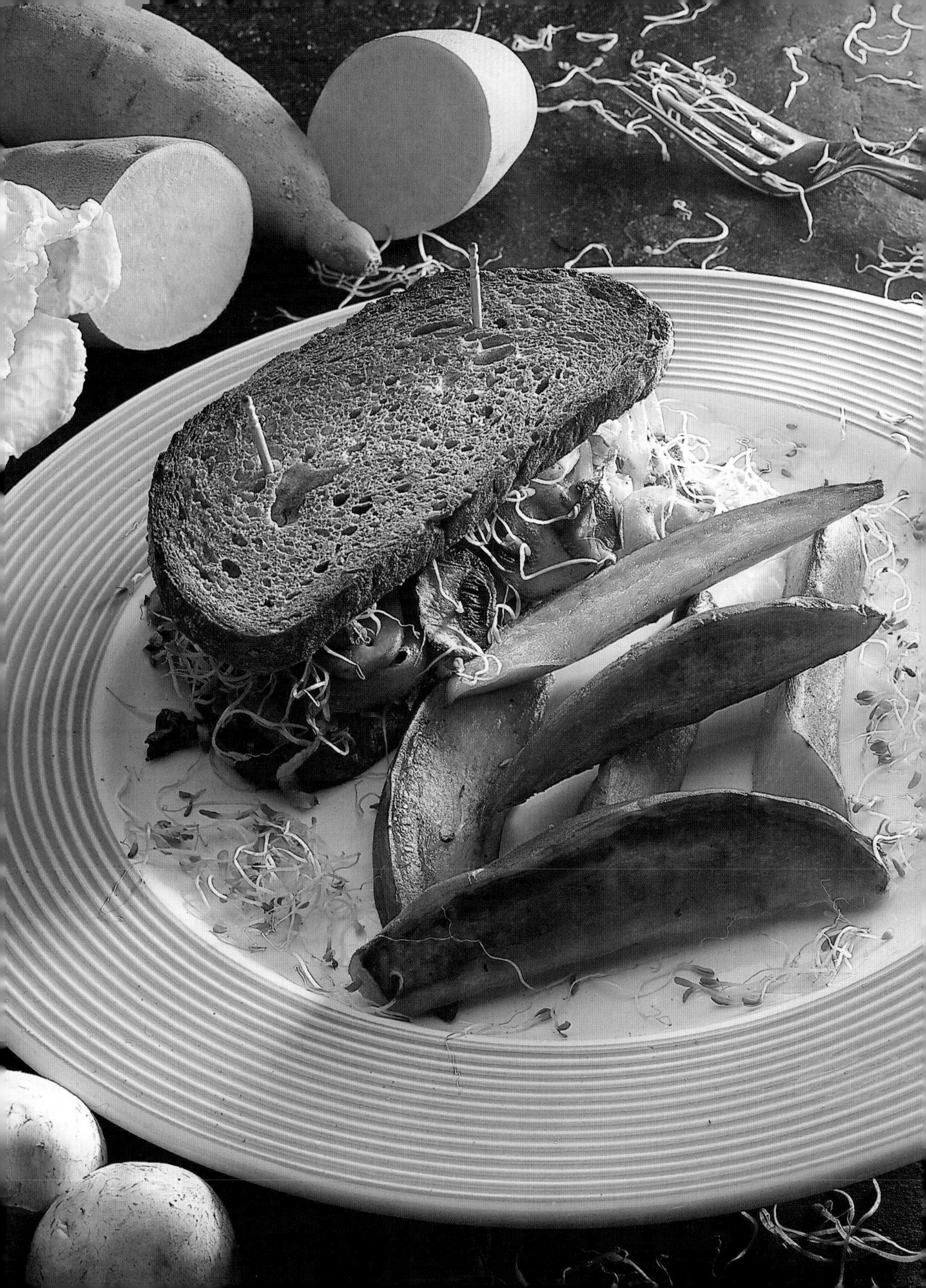

Currant Rice with Curried Vegetables

Brussels sprouts, cauliflower and broccoli belong to the cabbage family, and all are excellent sources of vitamin C and good sources of fiber and B vitamins.

- **⅛ cup** (50 g) **sun-dried currants or cranberries**
- **1 cup** (250 g) **organic long-grain brown rice**
- **1 cup** (250 g) **carrots, sliced diagonally 1"** (2.5 cm) **long and ½"** (1 cm) **wide**
- **1 cup** (250 g) **celery, sliced diagonally 1"** (2.5 cm) **long and ½"** (1 cm) **wide**
- **1 cup** (250 g) **Brussels sprouts, quartered**
- **1 cup** (250 g) **cauliflower florets**
- **1 cup** (250 g) **broccoli florets**
- **2 tbsp extra-virgin olive oil**
- **½ white onion, diced**
- **2 cloves garlic, minced**
- **2 tsp Marsala curry powder**
- **Pinch chili flakes**
- **Sea salt to taste**
- **1 tbsp fresh cilantro, chopped**

Wash the currants and soak them in water for 10 minutes. Drain and set aside.

In the meantime, bring the rice and 2 cups of water to a boil in a medium-size pot (covered) then reduce the heat to simmer. When the water is almost completely absorbed, add the currants, stir and continuing cooking until the water is fully absorbed. Remove the rice from the heat and keep warm.

In a large pot, bring 2 quarts (2 liters) of water to a boil and add the vegetables, individually, in the following order: carrots–cook for 3 minutes, then add celery, Brussels sprouts, cauliflower, and finish with the broccoli. From the time you add the carrots to the broccoli, the vegetables should cook for a total of 5 minutes at the most. Reserving the vegetable water, drain the vegetables and rinse them immediately with cold water. This action will halt cooking and lock in the vibrant taste, nutrients and color of the vegetables.

Heat the oil in a large pan over medium heat and sauté the onion and garlic until tender. Add ½ cup (125 ml) vegetable water and curry, then the vegetables. Cover and cook for 3 to 4 minutes or until the liquid is reduced by half. Add chili flakes, season with salt and garnish with cilantro.

Serve with the rice.

Serves 2

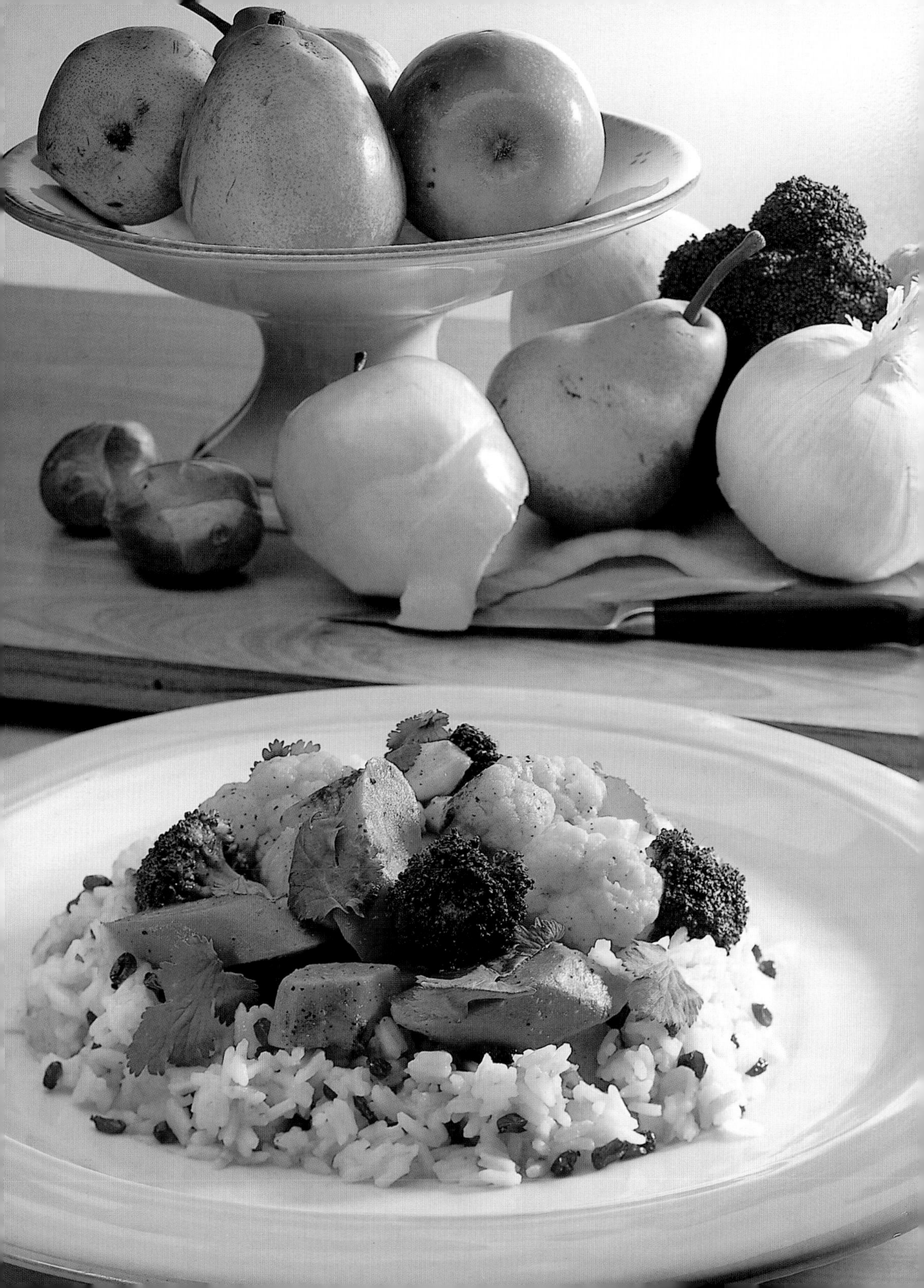

Vegetarian Paella

Mediterranean people are known to eat light and nutritious meals. This wholesome variation of the famous dish delivers the flavors of southern Spain without the risk of aggravating joint pain.

- **1 cup** (250 g) **carrots, sliced**
- **1 cup** (250 g) **Brussels sprouts, quartered**
- **1 cup** (250 g) **cauliflower florets**
- **1 cup** (250 g) **broccoli florets**
- **2 tbsp extra-virgin olive oil**
- ½ **cup** (125 g) **onion, diced**
- **3 cloves garlic, minced**
- **1 cup** (250 g) **organic long-grain brown rice**
- **1 tsp saffron**
- **2 tsp paprika**
- **1 bay leaf**
- **Sea salt to taste**
- **1 tsp lemon zest** (optional)
- **1 cup** (150 g) **mushrooms, sliced**
- ½ **cup** (125 g) **fresh or frozen green peas**
- **2 tbsp green onion, chopped for garnish**
- **1 tbsp fresh parsley, chopped for garnish**

In a large pot, bring 2 quarts (2 liters) of water to a boil and add the vegetables in the following order: carrots(cook for 3 minutes), then Brussels sprouts, cauliflower, and the broccoli last. From the time you add the carrots to the time you add the broccoli, the vegetables should cook for a total of 5 minutes at the most. Reserving the vegetable water, drain the vegetables and rinse them immediately with cold water.

In a large heavy skillet, heat oil over medium heat and sauté onion and garlic until tender. Add rice, sauté for an additional 2 minutes then add 1 cup (250 ml) reserved vegetable water, saffron, paprika, bay leaf, cayenne, salt and lemon zest. Stir, making sure all the rice is loose and does not stick to the pan. When ⅓ of the liquid is remaining, gradually add vegetables, starting with carrots, then Brussels sprouts, cauliflower, broccoli, mushrooms, and ending with peas. Cook for 10 to 12 minutes or until the water is fully absorbed.

Garnish with green onion and parsley and serve immediately.

Serves 2

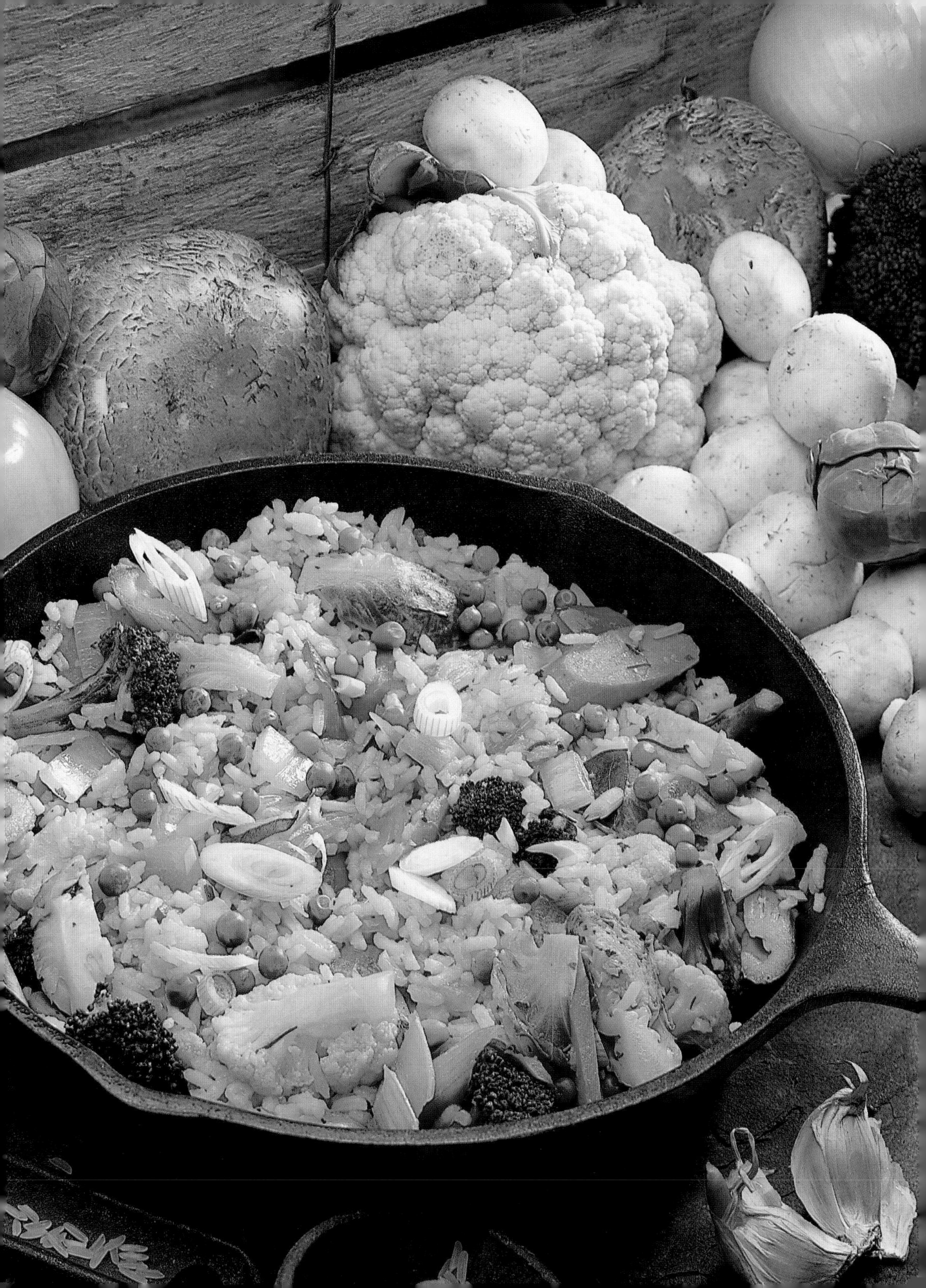

Panfried Polenta with Vegetable Ragout

Polenta:

2 cups (500 ml) **water**

Pinch sea salt

1 cup (250 g) **polenta** (coarse corn) **flour**

½ cup (120 g) **fresh corn kernels**

1 tbsp fresh oregano leaves

Sea salt to taste

2 tbsp + 4 tbsp extra-virgin olive oil

⅛ cup (30 g) **almond slices or sesame seeds**

¼ cup (60 g) **cornmeal**

Vegetable Ragout:

1 ½ tbsp cold-pressed olive oil

4 cloves garlic, sliced

1 cup (250 g) **carrots, sliced diagonally 1"** (2.5 cm) **wide**

1 cup (250 g) **celery, sliced diagonally 1"** (2.5 cm) **wide**

1 cup (250 g) **Brussels sprouts, cut in half**

1 cup (250 g) **turnip, peeled and sliced 1"** (2.5) **wide**

1 cup (250 g) **asparagus, cut 2"** (5 cm) **long**

To make the polenta, bring water and a pinch of salt to a boil in a medium-size pot. Slowly add polenta, stirring constantly with a wooden spoon for 7 to 10 minutes. Reduce heat to medium. Before the polenta starts to thicken, stir in corn and oregano. Season with salt and pepper. Add 2 tablespoons of olive oil and stir until thick. Remove from heat and let cool.

Mix together the polenta and almonds and shape the mixture into patties. Dip in cornmeal and panfry in 4 tablespoons of olive oil until both sides are golden brown. Keep the polenta warm in the oven.

To prepare the vegetables, bring 1 quart (1 liter) of water to a boil in a large pot and add the vegetables in the following order: carrots (cook for 3 minutes), then celery, Brussels sprouts, turnip, and asparagus last. From the time you add the carrots to the asparagus, the vegetables should cook for a total of 5 minutes at the most. Drain the vegetables and rinse them immediately with cold water.

In a large pan, heat oil over medium heat and sauté the garlic until slightly brown. Add vegetables and sauté for 3 to 4 minutes.

Place the polenta in the center of plates and pour vegetables around. Serve immediately.

Serves 2

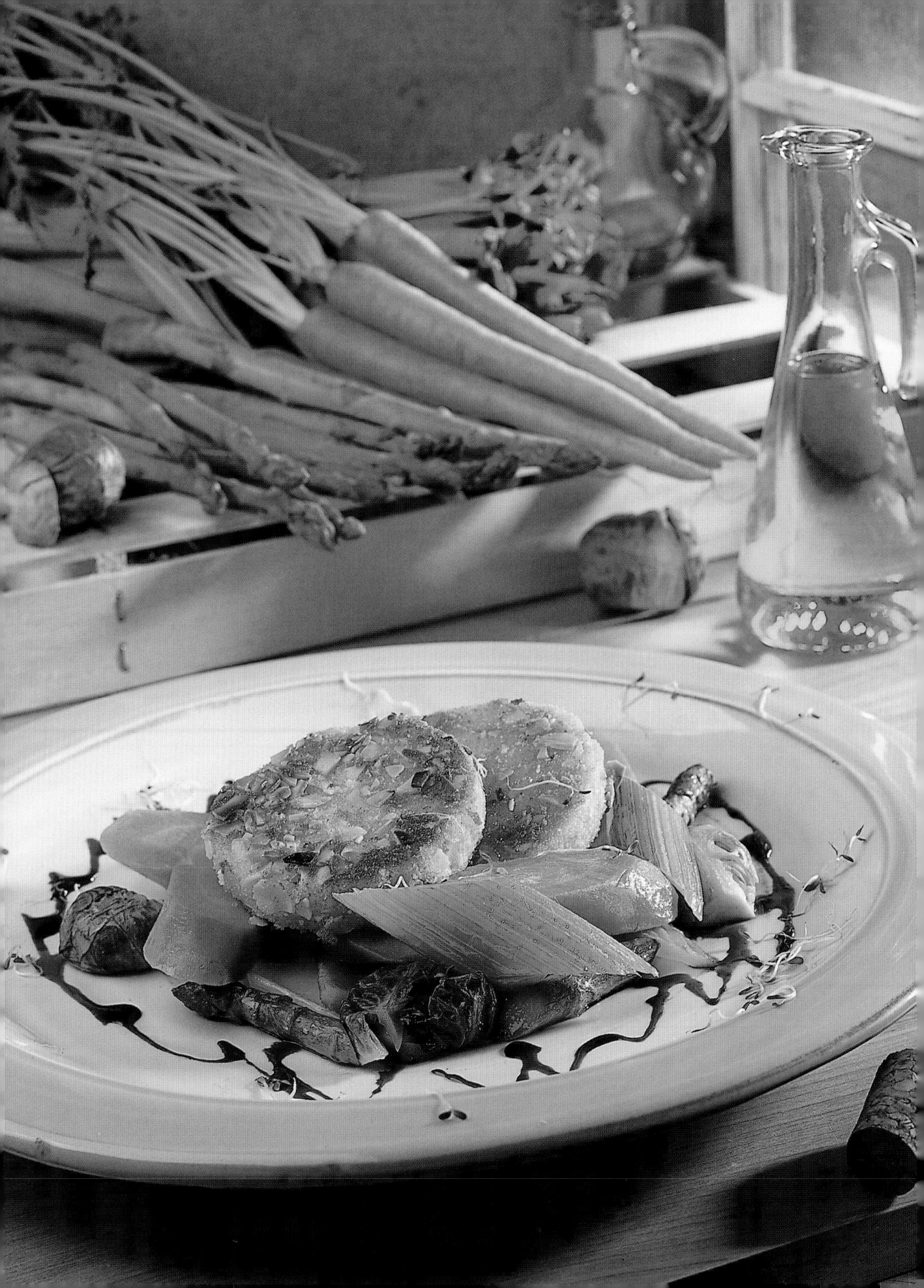

Apricot-Rice Patty with Fresh Fruit

Emphasizing raw fruit and vegetables in your daily meals will limit your calorie intake, and provide the nutrients needed for rebuilding joint cartilage and fluid.

1 cup (250 g) **short-grain brown rice**

2 cups (500 ml) **water**

½ cup (80 g) **dried apricots, sliced**

3 tbsp almonds, sliced

Pinch sea salt

Pinch ground cinnamon

Pinch ground nutmeg

2 tbsp extra-virgin olive oil

2 cups (450 g) **assorted fresh fruit, cut in wedges**

2 tsp freshly squeezed lemon juice

In a medium pot, bring water and rice to a boil, reduce heat to medium and cook until ⅔ liquid is evaporated. Add apricots and half the almonds. Season with salt, cinnamon and nutmeg and cook rice until water is fully absorbed. Remove from heat and let cool.

To make each patty, form 2 to 3 ounces (about ½ cup) of the rice mixture into a ball shape then press it flat. In a skillet, heat olive oil over medium heat and sauté both sides until golden brown.

Place the patties onto plates and arrange the fresh fruit around. Sprinkle remaining almonds over top and drizzle with lemon juice.

Serves 2

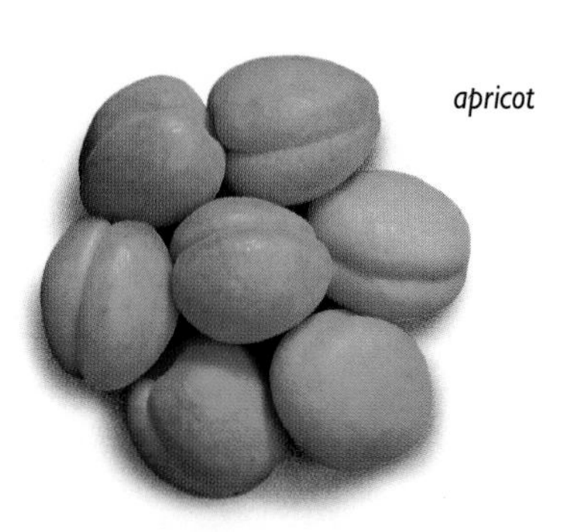

apricot

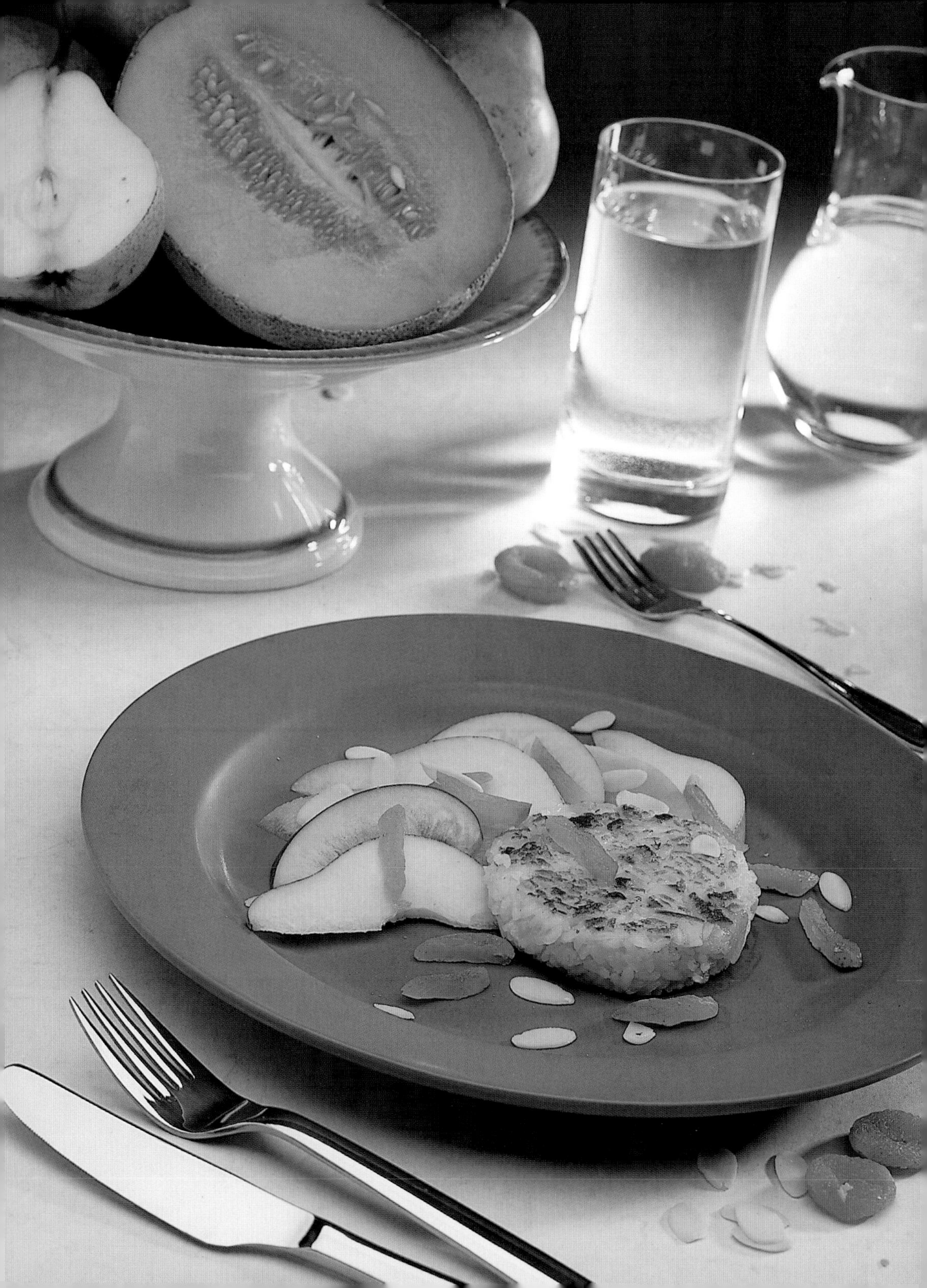

Cream of Wheat with Fresh Fruit

Melons are good sources of vitamins C and E, which work together to maintain and build cartilage. These vitamins also act as antioxidant protection against free-radical damage that contributes to arthritic inflammation. Health benefits aside, enjoying this wonderfully fresh breakfast is a great way to start the day.

1 cup (250 g) **organic cream of wheat**

1 ½ cups (375 ml) **water**

Zest of 1 lemon

1 tsp fresh mint, chopped (optional)

Pinch sea salt

1 tbsp coconut oil or butter

2 tsp ground cinnamon

1 small melon (such as cantaloupe or honeydew), **scooped into balls**

2 cups (450 g) **fresh mixed berries of your choice**

In a medium pot, bring the water to a boil and slowly add cream of wheat, stirring with a wooden spoon. Add 1 teaspoon of lemon zest and mint. Season with salt. Reduce heat to low and stir until mixture thickens to a batter-like consistency.

Pour the mixture into a glass pie dish until it's ½" (1 cm) high. Let cool until completely set. Remove from dish and cut into desired shape (use a cookie cutter, if you wish).

In a pan, heat oil over medium heat and sauté both sides until lightly golden and just warmed. Dust with cinnamon and place onto plates. Serve with fresh lemon zest and fruit.

Serves 2

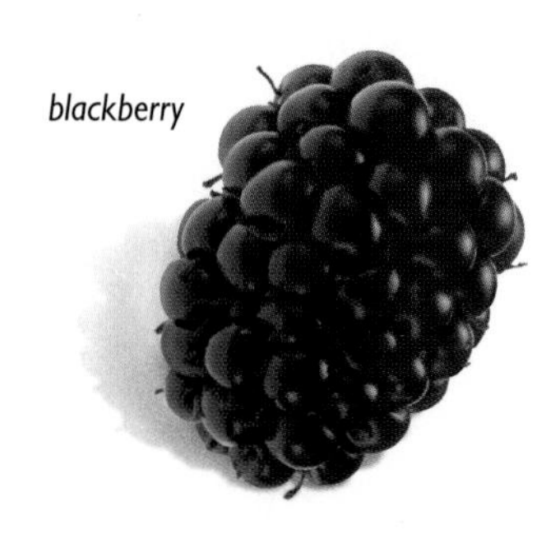

blackberry

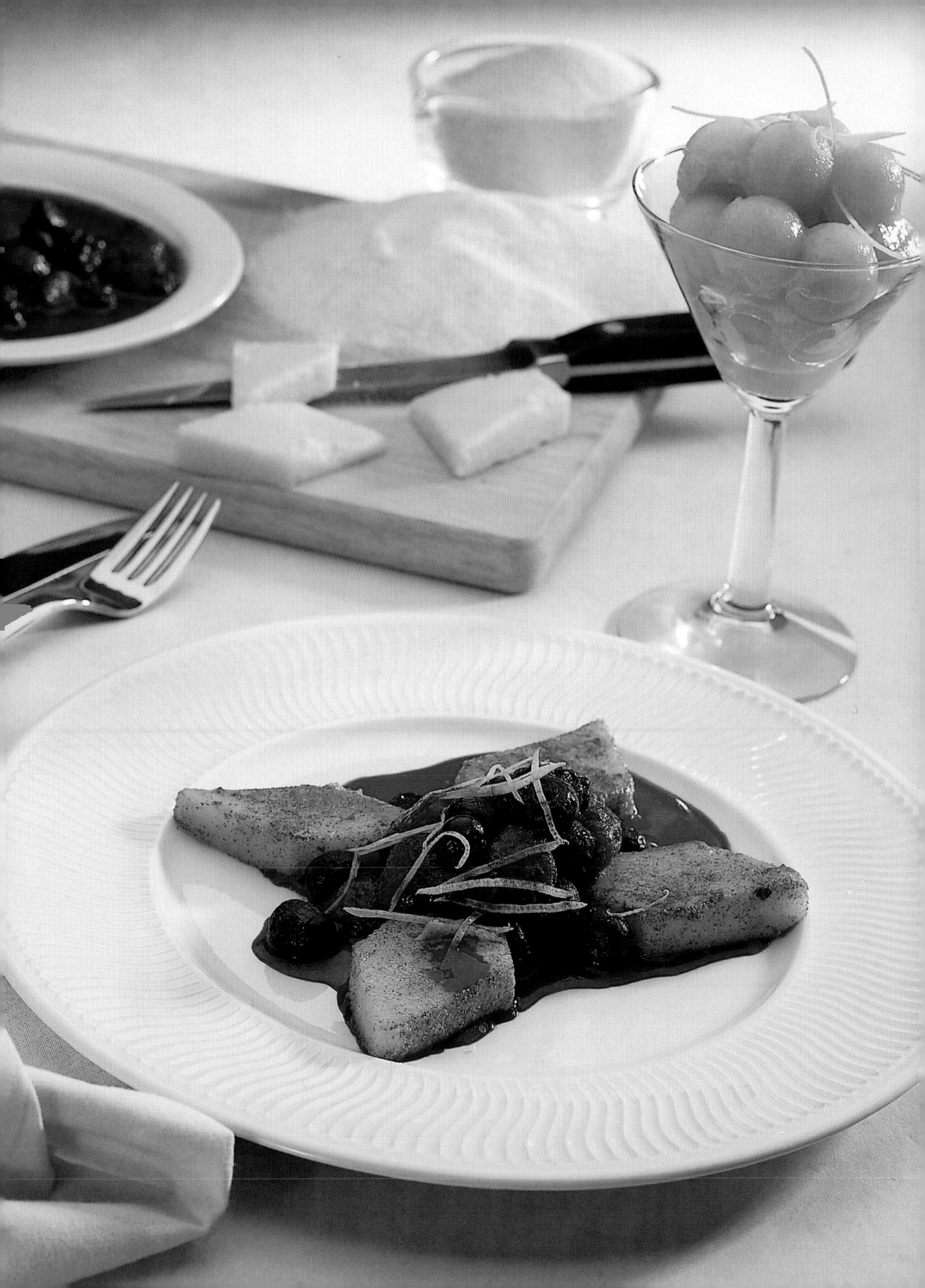

references

Bland, J.H., and S.M. Cooper. "Osteoarthritis: A review of the cell biology involved and evidence for reversibility." Semin. Arthritis Rheum. 14, no. 2 (1984): 106-33.

Gittleman, A.L. Guess What Came to Dinner: Parasites and your health. Garden City Park, NY: Avery, 1993.

Grennan, D.M., et al. "Serum copper and zinc in rheumatoid arthritis and osteoarthritis." New Zealand Medical Journal 91, no. 652 (1980): 47-50.

Hazenberg, M.P. "Intestinal floral, bacteria and arthritis: Why the joint?" Scandinavian Journal of Rheumatology 24 (1995): 207-211.

Jameson, S., et al. "Pain relief and selenium balance in patients with connective tissue disease and osteoarthritis." Nutr. Res. Suppl. 1 (1985): 391-97.

Jonas, W.B., et al. "The effect of niacinaminde on osteoarthritis: A pilot study." Inflammation Research 45 (1996): 330-34.

Krenner, J.M., et al. "Fish oil supplementation in active rheumatoid arthritis: A double-blinded, controlled, crossover study." Ann Intern Med. 106, no. 4 (1987): 497-503.

Lopez, Vaz A. "Double-blind clinical evaluation of the relative efficacy of ibuprofen and glucosamine sulfate in the management of osteoarthritis of the knee in out-patients." Curr. Med. Res. Opin. 8 (1982): 145-49.

Machtey, I., and L. Ouaknine. "Tocopherol in osteoarthritis: A controlled pilot study." Journal of the American Geriatric Society 26 (1978): 328.

McAlindon, Timothy E., et al. "Do antioxidant micronutrients protect against the development and progression of knee osteoarthritis?" Arthritis and Rheumatism 39, no. 4 (1996): 648-56.

Murray, Michael T. Natural Alternatives to Over-the-Counter and Prescription Drugs. New York: William Morrow and Company, 1994.

Stammers, T., et al. "Fish oil in osteoarthritis." Lancet 2 (1989): 503.

Theodosakis, Jason. The Arthritis Cure: The medical miracle that can halt, reverse and may even cure osteoarthritis. St. Martin's Press, 1996.

2

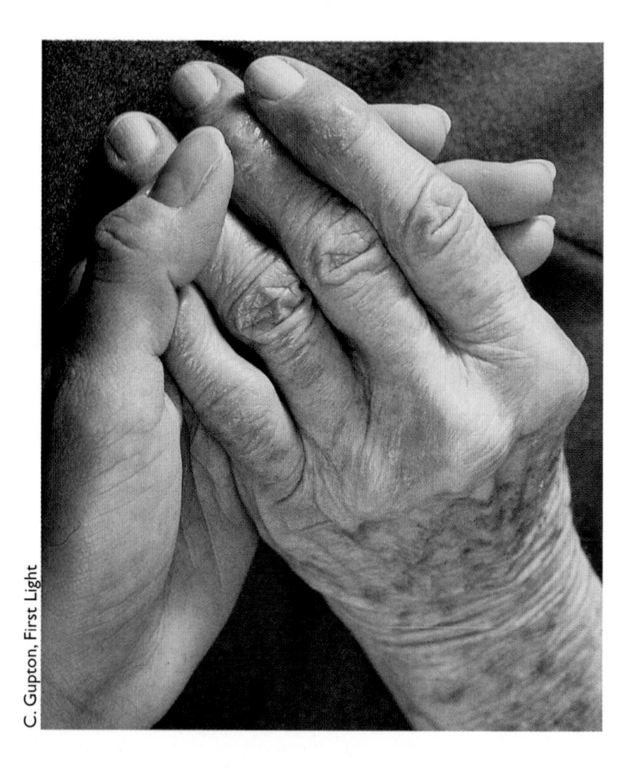

C. Gupton, First Light

sources

For herbal products and natural oils:
Flora Manufacturing & Distributing Ltd.
7400 Fraser Park Drive, Burnaby, BC
V5J 5B9 Canada
604-436-6000
1-888-436-6697 (Product Information)
www.florahealth.com

Flora Inc.
PO Box 73, 805 East Badger
Lynden WA 98264 USA
360-354-2110

For glucosamine sulfate and cod liver oil:
Natural Factors Nutritional Products Ltd.
1550 United Boulevard, Coquitlam, BC
V3K 6Y7 Canada
604-777-1757
1-800-663-8900 (Canada)
1-800-322-8704 (US)
www.naturalfactors.com

For hemp oil:
Hempola
2133 Forbes Road, RR#1 Barrie, ON
L4M 4Y8 Canada
705-730-0405
1-800-240-9215
www.hempola.com

For hemp foods and oils:
Manitoba Harvest Hemp Foods & Oils
c/o Fresh Hemp Foods Ltd.
#15-2166 Notre Dame Ave, Winnipeg, MB
R3H 0K2 Canada
1-800-665-4367
www.hemperor.com

First published in 2000 by
alive books
7436 Fraser Park Drive
Burnaby BC V5J 5B9
(604) 435–1919
1-800–661–0303

6th Printing - November 2006

Book Design:
Liza Novecoski
Artwork:
Terence Yeung
Raymond Cheung
Food Styling:
Fred Edrissi
Photography:
Edmond Fong (recipe photos)
Siegfried Gursche
Photo Editing:
Sabine Edrissi-Bredenbrock
Editing:
Sandra Tonn
Marian MacLean

Canadian Cataloguing in Publication Data

Rona MD, Zoltan
Osteoarthritis

(*alive* natural health guides, 16
ISSN 1490-6503)
ISBN 1-55312-013-2

Printed in Canada